2nd Edition

EMT EMERGENCY MEDICAL TECHNICIAN
CRASH COURSE®

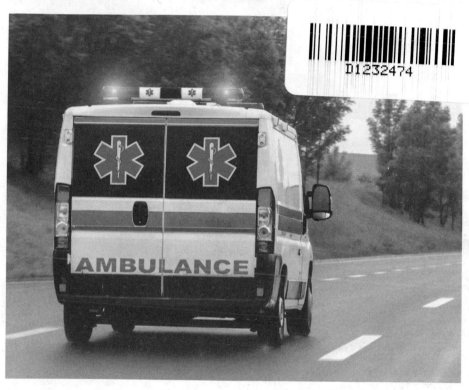

Chris Coughlin, NREMT-P, Ph.D.

Research & Education Association
Visit our website at: www.rea.com

Research & Education Association
61 Ethel Road West
Piscataway, New Jersey 08854
Email: info@rea.com

EMT CRASH COURSE®, 2ND EDITION

Copyright © 2018 by Research & Education Association, Inc.

Prior edition copyright © 2012 by Research & Education Association, Inc. All rights reserved. No part of this book may be reproduced in any form without permission of the publisher.

Printed in the United States of America

Library of Congress Control Number 2017951969

ISBN-13: 978-0-7386-1235-5
ISBN-10: 0-7386-1235-9

LIMIT OF LIABILITY/DISCLAIMER OF WARRANTY: Publication of this work is for the purpose of test preparation and related use and subjects as set forth herein. While every effort has been made to achieve a work of high quality, neither Research & Education Association, Inc., nor the authors and other contributors of this work guarantee the accuracy or completeness of or assume any liability in connection with the information and opinions contained herein and in REA's companion software and/or online materials. REA and the authors and other contributors shall in no event be liable for any personal injury, property or other damages of any nature whatsoever, whether special, indirect, consequential or compensatory, directly or indirectly resulting from the publication, use or reliance upon this work.

Cover image: © iStockphoto.com/OgnjenO

All trademarks cited in this publication are the property of their respective owners.

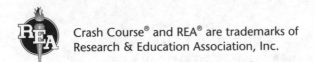

Crash Course® and REA® are trademarks of Research & Education Association, Inc.

EMT CRASH COURSE
TABLE OF CONTENTS

PART I   Introduction

PART II   Preparing to Become an EMT
Review plus end-of-chapter practice

PART III

Airway, Pharmacology, and Patient Assessment
Review plus end-of-chapter practice

PART IV

Shock, Resuscitation and Medical Emergencies
Review plus end-of-chapter practice

PART V

Trauma and Environmental Emergencies
Review plus end-of-chapter practice

PART VI

Special Patient Populations
Review plus end-of-chapter practice

PART VII

EMS Operations
Review plus end-of-chapter practice

PART VIII

The Practical Exam

A NOTE FROM OUR AUTHOR

It is impractical to try and learn every fact or concept in an EMS textbook. An EMS student must be able to distinguish the "must know" from the rest of the material presented. That's what this book does: it emphasizes the "must know" content. This *Crash Course* is unique because it's designed for those who are one test away from direct patient care in potentially dangerous circumstances.

This publication is not a substitute for a well-written textbook or participation in a high-quality EMS training program, but rather as a bridge between your training and your certification exam. This book helps you focus on the knowledge necessary to pass the NREMT certification exam and function competently as an EMT.

In EMT class, students take a test after the lesson. When you are an EMS provider, the test comes unannounced and the lesson is learned afterward. When you are not prepared for class, you risk a poor grade. When you are not prepared on the street, the patient pays the price.

As you work your way through this book, imagine yourself certified, hired, and on duty for your very first shift:

You have just been dispatched to the community pool. There are reports of a fire in a storage room near the pool with a number of people fleeing the area. The dispatcher tells you a lifeguard is performing CPR on a child pulled from the water during the evacuation.

> You don't know if you will be the first EMS unit on the scene . . .

> You don't know what was in the storage room or what hazards await you . . .

> You don't know how many patients are waiting for your help, or what might be wrong with them . . .

> You don't know if you will be caring for the pediatric drowning victim or other patients . . .

With this scenario in mind, read through this book and ask yourself, "What do I really need to know to handle this call?"

Study hard and good luck on your certification exam.

Be safe!

Chris Coughlin, NREMT-P, Ph.D.

ABOUT OUR BOOK

REA's *EMT Crash Course* is designed for the last-minute studier or any prospective Emergency Medical Technician who wants a quick refresher before taking the NREMT Certification Exam. Our *Crash Course* will show you how to study efficiently and strategically, so you can pass your exam.

Written by a veteran EMS Program Director and NREMT paramedic, REA's *EMT Crash Course* gives you a review specifically targeted to what you really need to know to ace the exam.

- **Parts I and II** offer tips for succeeding on the exam, along with an overview of the EMT's role and the anatomy of the human body.

- **Parts III, IV, and V** cover patient assessment, resuscitation, trauma, and medical and environmental emergencies.

- **Part VI** explains special patient care, including pediatric and geriatric patients.

- **Part VII** reviews EMS operations, such as ambulance and air medical operations.

- **Part VIII** discusses how to prepare for the practical exam as well as what to do after you pass you exam.

- **End-of-chapter practice questions** help you review what you've learned.

- **EMT Glossary** includes 400 study terms you need to know to ace the exam. Go to *www.rea.com/emt* to download the list.

ABOUT OUR PRACTICE EXAM

Are you ready for the exam? Find out by taking **REA's online practice exam** available at *www.rea.com/emt*. This true-to-format practice test features automatic scoring and detailed explanations of all answers. It will help you identify your strengths and weaknesses so you'll be ready on exam day.

Good luck on your EMT exam!

ABOUT OUR AUTHOR

Dr. Chris Coughlin is the EMS Program Director for Glendale Community College in Glendale, Arizona. Dr. Coughlin has been an NREMT paramedic since 1991 and was one of the first 850 nationally certified flight paramedics (FP-C) in the United States.

Dr. Coughlin earned his AAS in Advanced Emergency Medical Technology from Glendale Community College; his B.A. in Adult Education from Ottawa University, Phoenix, Arizona; his M.Ed. in Educational Leadership from Northern Arizona University, Flagstaff, Arizona, and his Ph.D. in Professional Studies from Capella University, Minneapolis, Minnesota.

Dr. Coughlin welcomes correspondence at: chris.coughlin@gcmail.maricopa.edu.

AUTHOR DEDICATION AND ACKNOWLEDGMENTS

Dedicated to all U.S. military combat medics.

Special thanks to the instructors of the Basic Medical Technician Corpsmen Program, Medical Education & Training Campus, Fort Sam Houston, San Antonio, Texas.

Special thanks also to Sue Darroch-Wienberg, NREMT, for her critical eye, expertise, and attention to detail.

ACKNOWLEDGMENTS

In addition to our author, we would like to thank Larry B. Kling, Vice President, Editorial, for his overall guidance, which brought this publication to completion; Pam Weston, Publisher, for setting the quality standards for production integrity and managing the publication to completion; Diane Goldschmidt, Managing Editor, for editorial project management; and Alice Leonard, Senior Editor, for preflight editorial review.

We also extend our special thanks to Jeffrey Lindsey for his technical review of the manuscript, Caroline Duffy for copyediting, and Kathy Caratozzolo of Caragraphics for typesetting this edition.

PART I

INTRODUCTION

Preparing for Success on the NREMT Certification Exam

Serving the public as an Emergency Medical Technician (EMT) is among today's most rewarding careers. The overwhelming majority of states in the U.S. require that you pass the National Registry of Emergency Medical Technicians (NREMT) exam to become certified and work as an EMT. Certification through the NREMT indicates that you have demonstrated entry-level competency as an EMT.

The NREMT certification exam is a "pass/fail" test. Its purpose is not to identify who is the "best," but to identify who is "competent." Your future patients don't care what you scored on your certification exam. They care about receiving competent and compassionate care for themselves and those they care about. This *Crash Course* gives you the essential information you need to prepare for the NREMT certification exam.

I. THE EXAM

The NREMT exam is a computer-adaptive test (CAT). The test tailors itself to your individual abilities. The exam delivers questions one at a time and the questions are *not* randomly chosen. While you are taking the test, the software that drives the test is estimating your ability level. The ability estimate gets more and more precise as the exam progresses. The exam ends when there is a 95% certainty that your demonstrated competency is above or below the passing standard.

The NREMT complies with the Americans with Disabilities Act (ADA) of 1990 and offers reasonable accommodations for individuals with disabilities.

II. TOPICS COVERED ON THE EXAM

Your NREMT exam will most likely have at least 70 and no more than 120 questions. You will have two hours to complete the test. Less than 1% of candidates are unable to finish the exam in the time allowed. Take the time to read every question carefully. All of the questions will be multiple-choice and each question will have 4 answer choices. You need to choose the "best" answer for the question posed.

The exam will broadly cover the content of the current National EMS Education Standards (NEMSES) and the current *American Heart Association's Guidelines for Cardiopulmonary Resuscitation and Emergency Cardiovascular Care.* Correct answers are based on national standards, not local or state protocols. The exam emphasizes questions about what an EMT should do in the field, so you should expect a lot of scenario-based questions.

Topics will include airway, oxygenation, ventilation, cardiology, resuscitation, stroke, trauma, medical emergencies, obstetrics, gynecology, and EMS operations. Here are the percentages for the topics found on the exam.

NREMT Exam Topics	% of Test by Topic
Airway and ventilation	18%–22%
Cardiology, resuscitation, stroke	20%–24%
Trauma	14%–18%
Medical and OB/GYN	27%–31%
EMS operations	10%–14%

Source: https://www.nremt.org/rwd/public/document/cognitive-exam

For all but EMS operations, 85% of the questions relate to adult patients and 15% relate to pediatric patients. Although not separate categories, topics such as patient assessment, anatomy and physiology, pediatric emergencies, and safety will be emphasized throughout the test.

III. SCORING

Typically, you can retrieve your score from the NREMT website 24 hours after you complete the exam. If you fail the exam, the NREMT will provide some detailed information about your performance on each of the exam categories. Candidates must wait at least 14 days before taking the test again.

IV. STANDARDS

Like the NREMT certification exam, the information in this publication is based on the 2009 National EMS Education Standards and the 2010 *American Heart Association's Guidelines for Cardiopulmonary Resuscitation and Emergency Cardiovascular Care*. This *Crash Course* will help you become familiar with these standards before taking the certification exam; however, you should not rely on any one resource to prepare for the exam. For more information about the 2009 NEMSES, visit *www.ems. gov/education/nationalstandardandncs.html*. For more information about the current *American Heart Association's Guidelines,* visit *https://eccguide-lines.heart.org/index.php/circulation/cpr-ecc-guidelines-2/*.

V. GENERAL TEST-TAKING TIPS & STRATEGIES

- Try to take your NREMT exam soon after finishing your EMT course. The longer you wait to take the exam, the less likely you are to pass.

- Study regularly over an extended period before the test. Don't cram. Your preparation should end (not begin) the day before the test.

- Avoid caffeine, energy drinks, excess sugar, etc. These will not improve your performance or steady your nerves.

- Know exactly where the test center is and plan to arrive a few minutes early. Remember, you must have an appointment to take the test. Bring two forms of photo ID.

- Dress comfortably so you are not distracted by being too hot or too cold while taking the test.

VI. DURING THE TEST

- You *cannot* skip a question or come back to it later. You must answer each question before the next one will be provided.

- Read the whole question thoroughly at least a couple of times and formulate the answer in your head *before* you look at the answer choices. If you see a similar answer choice, that's probably the correct response.

- There are four answer choices. Two of them can often be eliminated after reading the question thoroughly. There is only one "best" answer.

- When you get stuck, look for key words in the question and re-read the answer choices. When in doubt, lean towards the more aggressive treatment. For example, if you are not sure whether you should ventilate the patient or just administer oxygen, choose to ventilate.

- Do *not* complicate scenario-based questions. Do not bring elements into the questions that are not there.

- Relax! Remember, everyone is going to feel like the test is extremely challenging. Everyone is going to miss a lot of questions. This does NOT mean you are failing.

VII. EXAMPLE ITEMS

Visit the NREMT website at *https://www.nremt.org/rwd/public/document/cognitive-exam.* You will be able to view three practice questions that will give you an idea of what to expect on the exam. According to the NREMT, the difficulty levels of these questions are either at or above the passing standard. If you find these questions to be easy, that's a great sign! If not, don't worry. We're just getting started.

PART II
PREPARING TO BECOME AN EMT

The Emergency Medical Services System:
History, Public Health, and the EMT's Role

I. THE EMERGENCY MEDICAL SERVICES (EMS) SYSTEM

A. EMS is a coordinated network of personnel and resources designed to provide emergency medical care and, when indicated, transport patients to an appropriate higher level of care.

B. EMS is also expected to serve a role in the larger public health system through public education and prevention efforts.

II. HISTORY OF THE EMS SYSTEM

A. The modern EMS system has its origins in funeral homes, which often operated ambulances. This former practice produced an environment in which funeral home operators were serving competing business interests, and patients received little trained care until they arrived at the hospital.

B. EMS is still an evolving profession, younger than many other health-care professions, such as nursing.

C. The 1960s

   1. In 1966, a paper titled *Accidental Death and Disability: The Neglected Disease of Modern Society* is published by the National Academy of Sciences. This paper is widely known in the EMS profession as the "White Paper."

      i.   The White Paper is widely considered the birth of modern EMS. It spotlighted inadequacies of prehospital care in the United States, particularly related to trauma.

D. The 1970s

1. Early in the decade, the U.S. Department of Transportation (DOT) develops the first EMT National Standard Curriculum (NSC).

2. The first EMT textbook is published.

3. Later in the decade, the DOT also publishes the first paramedic NSC.

E. The 1980s

1. The American Heart Association (AHA) dramatically increases its emphasis on cardiovascular disease prevention, science, and education.

2. Additional levels of training are added to the existing EMT and paramedic curriculum.

3. Despite advances, the scope of practice for various levels of training lacks unity from state to state.

F. The 1990s

1. The National Registry of Emergency Medical Technicians (NREMT) advocates for a national training curriculum.

2. The National Highway Transportation Safety Administration (NHTSA) begins work on the *EMS Agenda for the Future* document.

3. Public access defibrillation and layperson training on the use of automated external defibrillators (AEDs) sweeps across the country. This has a significant impact on survival of out-of-hospital cardiac arrest.

G. The 2000s

1. In line with the *EMS Agenda for the Future,* the NHTSA identifies universal knowledge and skills for EMS professionals through the new National EMS Education Standards (NEMSES).

   i. The new NEMSES replace the previous National Standard Curricula.

   ii. Four new levels of EMS licensure/certification are created: Emergency Medical Responder, Emergency Medical Technician, Advanced Emergency Medical Technician, and Paramedic.

Author's Note: For more on the history of EMS, I recommend watching the DVD *Making A Difference: The History of Modern EMS* Version 2.0, narrated by Jim Page, founder of Jems Communications.

III. COMPONENTS OF THE EMS SYSTEM

A. Public access: refers to how the public accesses the EMS system

B. Clinical care: outlines the scope of practice and associated equipment

C. Medical direction: physician oversight of patient care

D. Integrated health services: prehospital service providers work cooperatively with hospital personnel to ensure continuity of care

E. Information systems: the information technology component of the EMS system

F. Prevention: the EMS system's role in preventing injury and illness

G. Research: the move toward EMS care based on evidence-based medicine

H. Communications: communication systems used to activate EMS system, dispatch responders, and communicate with medical direction

I. Human resources: attempts to professionalize EMS occupations

J. Legislation and regulation: ensures the EMS system conforms to various local, state, and federal requirements

K. Evaluation: the quality improvement component of the EMS system

L. Finance: addresses the funding sources of the EMS system

M. Public education: focuses on the EMS system's role in the larger public health system

N. Education systems: addresses the quality of EMS training

IV. ACCESSING THE EMS SYSTEM

A. 911 and non-911 Access

1. Most 911 systems are "enhanced," allowing for automatic number and location identification by the dispatcher.

2. Many EMS systems use specially trained Emergency Medical Dispatchers (EMDs) able to give medical instructions to callers.

3. Cell-phone 911 calls and an increasing number of residences without landlines present new challenges for accessing the EMS system or confirming the location of the incident.

V. LEVELS OF TRAINING

A. **Emergency Medical Responder (EMR):** provides basic, immediate care including bleeding control, CPR, AED, and emergency childbirth. (Previously known as First Responder.)

B. **Emergency Medical Technician (EMT):** includes all EMR skills, advanced oxygen and ventilation skills, pulse oximetry, noninvasive blood pressure (BP) monitoring, and administration of certain medications. (Previously known as EMT-Basic.)

C. **Advanced Emergency Medical Technician (AEMT):** includes all EMT skills, advanced airway devices, intravenous and intraosseous access, blood glucose monitoring, and administration of additional medications.

D. **Paramedic:** includes all preceding training levels, advanced assessment and management skills, various invasive skills, and extensive pharmacology interventions. This is the highest level of prehospital care outlined in the National EMS Education Standards.

Paramedic

AEMT skills plus:
BiPAP/CPAP
Needle decompression
Percutaneous
   cricothyrotomy
$ETCO_2$/capnography
NG/OG tube
Intubaiton
Direct laryngoscopy
PEEP
ECG interpretation
Manual defibrillation/
   cardioversion
Transcutaneous external
   pacing
Extensive medication
   administration
Thrombolytic therapy

AEMT

EMT skills plus:
Multilumen airways
Blood glucose
   monitoring
IV/IO insertion
Medication
   administration

EMT

EMT skills plus:
Humidified oxygen
Venturi mask
Automated transport
   ventilators
Nasal airways
Pulse oximetry
Auto BP
Assisted medications
Spinal immobilization
Splinting
Tourniquet
MAST/PASG
Mechanical CPR
Assisted complicated
   childbirth

EMR

CPR, AED
Oral airways
Airway obstruction
Manual airway
   techniques
BVM ventilation
Oxygen therapy
Airway suctioning
Manual BP
Auto injector
Bleeding control
Assisted childbirth

VI. DESTINATION FACILITIES

A. EMTs routinely transport patients to a local medical emergency department (ED) based on the chief complaint or patient request.

B. In certain situations, patients may be transported to a specialty facility.

1. Stroke center: provides rapid specialized care for stroke patients

2. Cardiac center: equipped to provide rapid intervention for cardiac emergencies

3. Trauma center: capable of providing rapid surgical intervention

4. Behavioral center: specializes in management of behavioral emergencies

5. Pediatric center: provides specialty pediatric care

6. Obstetric center: equipped for high-risk obstetrical patients

7. Poison center: provides specialized care for toxicology patients

VII. EMT ROLES AND RESPONSIBILITIES

A. Equipment preparedness

B. Emergency vehicle operations

C. Establish, maintain scene safety

D. Patient assessment and treatment

E. Lifting and moving

F. Strong verbal and written communication skills

G. Patient advocacy

H. Professional development

I. Quality improvement

J. Illness and injury prevention

K. Maintain certification/licensure

VIII. PATIENT SAFETY

A. EMTs routinely participate in activities that are "high risk" for the patient. These activities require adequate training, focus, and attention to detail.

1. Transfer of patient care. This includes moving the patient from one stretcher to another and providing all necessary information to allow continuity of care.

2. Lifting and moving patients. Patients often incur avoidable injuries while being lifted or moved by EMS providers. This includes moving patients by wheeled stretcher and during loading and unloading of patients.

3. Transporting the patient in an ambulance. All occupants in the back of an ambulance are at risk of injury (especially unrestrained EMS providers). Safety is the priority during transport, not speed.

4. Spinal precautions. Patients can suffer devastating injuries if spinal precautions are not taken when indicated, or are not performed competently. Patients can also suffer unnecessarily if they are placed in spinal precautions when not indicated.

5. Administration of medications. Medication errors are frighteningly common.

B. Errors by EMS providers that result in patient injury are usually due to

1. failure to perform skills adequately.

2. lack of knowledge leading to poor decision making.

3. failure to follow established protocols.

C. Preventing Errors

1. Make sure you understand your protocols and follow them.

2. Provide the best possible environment to assess and manage patients; for example, ensure adequate lighting, minimize distractions, etc.

3. When in doubt, consult your partner, Advanced Life Support (ALS) providers, or medical direction.

IX. PROFESSIONAL ATTRIBUTES

A. Professional appearance

B. Competent knowledge, skills

C. Physical capability

D. Leadership skills

E. High ethical standards

F. Emotional stability

G. Critical/adaptive thinking skills

H. Effective listener

I. Ability to function in team environment

X. MEDICAL DIRECTION

A. The medical director is a physician responsible for providing medical oversight.

B. Online medical direction: direct contact between the physician and EMT via phone or radio.

C. Offline medical direction: written guidelines and protocols.

D. The medical director oversees quality improvement.

XI. QUALITY IMPROVEMENT (QI)

A. Also called continuous quality improvement (CQI).

B. Continuous audit and review of all aspects of the EMS system to identify areas of improvement.

XII. PUBLIC HEALTH

A. EMS providers are part of the larger public health system.

B. The public health system is responsible for the overall health of the entire population.

C. Examples of the EMS system's participation in public health efforts may include immunization clinics, prevention education, safety, wellness events, and public CPR training.

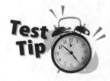

Your preparation for the national certification exam should have two distinct components:

1. Assemble the information you plan to learn before taking the exam.

   i. Create flashcards after reviewing each chapter in this book—each flashcard should contain a reasonable amount of information.

2. Learn the information you have assembled. Keep a few flashcards with you at all times and review them several times each day.

PRACTICE QUESTIONS

1. Which of the following is widely considered to mark the beginning of the modern EMS system?

   A. A paper titled *Accidental Death and Disability: The Neglected Disease of Modern Society*.

   B. The current National EMS Education Standards.

   C. The creation of the American Heart Association.

   D. A paper called the *EMS Agenda for the Future*.

2. EMS care today is based on

   A. what has been done in the past.

   B. whatever physicians recommend.

   C. evidence-based medicine.

   D. the original National Standard Curriculum.

3. Which of the following describes the EMT level of training?

   A. provides basic, immediate care including bleeding control, CPR, AED, and emergency childbirth

   B. includes oxygen and ventilation skills, pulse oximetry, and administration of certain medications

   C. includes advanced assessment and management skills, various invasive skills, and extensive pharmacology interventions

   D. includes advanced airway devices, intravenous and intraosseous access, and blood glucose monitoring

4. EMT roles and responsibilities include

   A. strong written and verbal communication skills.

   B. the ability to establish intraosseous access.

   C. initial investigation at a crime scene.

   D. swift water rescue operations.

5. Which of the following EMT activities is considered high risk for the patient?

   A. assessment of vital signs

   B. obtaining a blood glucose test

   C. requesting permission to treat

   D. transferring patient care

ANSWERS

1. **A.**

   This document is also known as the "White Paper" and precedes the current NEMSES and the *EMS Agenda for the Future*. The AHA did not establish the modern EMS system. (Note that the correct answer is much longer than the other answer choices. This is often a clue for choosing the correct answer. However, the NREMT knows this and strives to make all answer choices on their tests similar in length.)

2. **C.**

   EMS care today is based on evidence-based medicine, not what has been done in the past or what others recommend.

3. **B.**

   Option A describes the EMR level training. Option C describes paramedic training and option D describes AEMT levels of training.

4. **A.**

   The other answer choices are *not* typically roles and responsibilities of the EMT.

5. **D.**

   Transfer of care is one of five high-risk activities listed in this chapter. During transfer of care, the patient must be safely moved from one stretcher to another along with all necessary information related to the patient in order to allow continuity of care.

EMT Safety and Wellness/ Lifting and Moving/ Patient Restraint

I. SCENE SAFETY

A. The EMT's first priority is always his or her own safety. This will not change. This concept is a high priority on the certification exam. *Scene safety is always the top priority!*

B. The EMT's safety priorities after personal safety are for his/her partner(s), patients, and bystanders.

C. Maintaining scene safety includes addressing scene-specific hazards, appropriate infection control precautions, and safe lifting and moving techniques.

II. EMT WELLNESS

A. Physical Well-Being. Job tasks require that EMTs maintain a certain level of physical conditioning, get adequate sleep, and eat a healthy diet.

B. Mental Well-Being. EMTs must recognize that stress is an inevitable consequence of the profession. EMTs must anticipate stress and develop a healthy plan to help manage it.

1. Types of stress

   i. Acute stress: an immediate physiological and psychological reaction to a specific event. The event triggers the body's "fight or flight" response.

   ii. Delayed stress: a stress reaction that develops after the stressful event. It does not interfere with the EMT's ability to perform during the stressful event. Posttraumatic stress disorder (PTSD) is an example of delayed stress.

   iii. Cumulative stress: the result of exposure to stressful situations over a prolonged period of time. This leads to burnout for many EMTs.

2. Causes of stress

   i. Long hours, low pay, lack of sleep

   ii. Dangerous situations, exposure to death and dying

   iii. Challenging interactions with patients, family members, etc.

   iv. Working holidays, birthdays, anniversaries, etc.

   v. Nonemergency transports and aggressive system-status management

3. Managing stress

   i. Recognize signs of stress or burnout: anxiousness; irritability; headache; poor concentration; loss of appetite; difficulty sleeping; loss of interest in sex, hobbies, work, family, friends; increased use of alcohol or drugs.

   ii. Address modifiable risk factors for heart disease and stroke: tobacco use, hypertension, lack of exercise, and poor diet.

   iii. Find time for relaxing activities and interests; listen to the observations of family and friends. They know you best.

   iv. Balance the demands of your personal and professional life.

   v. Consider a change in your work environment, or get professional counseling.

   vi. Critical Incident Stress Management (CISM). CISM is a formalized process to help emergency workers deal with stress.

> ➤ Defusing sessions, when needed, are held within 4 hours of the incident.

> ➤ Debriefing sessions are held 24 to 72 hours after the incident.

> ➤ CISM teams consist of trained peer counselors and mental health experts.

> ➤ Participants can, but are not required to, share their feelings.

➤ CISM is meant to facilitate the process of dealing with critical incident stress. It is not used as a critique of patient care or any other type of performance evaluation.

➤ The information shared during a CISM session is confidential.

C. Emotional Demands of the EMS Profession

1. Routine exposure to death and dying

2. Encounters with patients in the various stages of grief

   i. Denial. The patient may experience a "not me" stage.

   ii. Anger. The patient may experience a "why me?" stage.

   iii. Bargaining. The patient may experience a "but I still need to . . . " stage.

   iv. Depression. The patient may experience a state of despair.

   v. Acceptance. The patient may come to accept death.

3. Interacting with the patient's family members during death and dying

   i. Show respect and empathy for patient and family.

   ii. Serve as a patient advocate.

   iii. Be supportive and keep the patient and family informed.

   iv. Do not use platitudes or offer false hope.

   v. Allow family to be with the patient whenever possible.

   vi. The family may need you even after there is nothing more you can do for the patient.

4. Routine exposure to high-stress situations, such as

   i. calls involving children or fellow emergency service workers.

   ii. violence, or significant traumatic injuries, such as burns.

   iii. frequent users of the EMS system.

   iv. patients who need more than the EMS system is able to provide.

   v. high call volume and sleep deprivation.

III. **EMTS AND INFECTIOUS DISEASES**

A. Infectious diseases are caused by an invading pathogen. Bacterial infections, such as strep throat, usually respond to prescription antibiotics. Viral infections, such as the flu, are resistant to antibiotics.

B. Diseases can be transmitted through direct person-to-person contact or indirect contact, such as touching a doorknob or telephone.

C. Standard Precautions

1. The Occupational Safety and Health Administration (OSHA) oversees regulations concerning workplace safety, including infectious disease precautions.

2. Employers provide the necessary equipment and implement and enforce infection control policies. They also provide mandatory training on infection control, exposure reporting, and blood-borne pathogens.

3. Employees are required to complete mandatory training and follow written infection control policies.

4. Standard precautions (formerly known as "universal precautions" or "body substance isolation precautions") are to be implemented for all patient contacts and are based on the assumption that all body fluids pose the risk of infection.

   i. Immediately report exposures to the designated infection control officer.

   ii. Handwashing is the single most important way to prevent the spread of infection. Hand sanitizers can be effective, but soap and water is preferred when available.

   iii. Personal protective equipment (PPE)

   ➤ PPE includes the equipment and supplies necessary to implement standard precautions for a specific patient encounter. PPE can differ from patient to patient based on the exposure risk.

   ➤ Minimum PPE. Gloves and eye protection should be used during any patient contact situation.

   ➤ Expanded PPE. Use disposable gown and mask for significant contact with any body fluid—for example, during childbirth. Use a high-efficiency particulate air

(HEPA) mask or N-95 respirator for suspected airborne disease exposure, such as tuberculosis.

iv. Additional infection control guidelines

➤ Contaminated medical waste should be enclosed in special "biohazard" bags and disposed of according to local and federal guidelines.

➤ Disposable supplies are intended for single patient use. They reduce the risk of exposure and are usually preferred to reusable equipment.

➤ Reusable equipment such as stretchers and BP cuffs must be properly cleaned with an approved disinfectant after every use.

➤ "Sharps" (needles, lancets, etc.) are placed in designated puncture-proof containers. Sharps should *not* be recapped before placing in an approved sharps container.

D. Recommended Immunizations and Vaccines

1. Regular TB testing (at least annually)

2. Hepatitis B vaccination series

3. Tetanus shot (every 10 years)

4. Flu vaccine (annual)

5. MMR vaccine: measles, mumps, rubella (as needed)

6. Varicella vaccine (as needed)

IV. PREVENTING WORK-RELATED INJURIES

A. Use the vehicle restraint system properly at all times, especially while attending to a patient during transport.

B. Hazardous Materials. Upon encountering a hazardous materials (hazmat) incident, the EMT should do the following:

1. Maintain a safe distance and attempt to keep others out.

2. Call for specially trained hazmat responders.

3. Look for placards without entering the scene, and utilize the *Emergency Response Guidebook* (ERG) to determine evacuation distance. (The ERG is required in all emergency vehicles.)

4. Do *not* enter a hazmat scene until cleared by hazmat specialists.

5. Do *not* begin emergency care until patients have been decontaminated or otherwise cleared by hazmat crews.

C. Crime Scenes

1. EMS providers should not enter a crime scene unless law enforcement has determined it is safe.

2. EMS providers may be advised to respond to the call but maintain a safe distance away until cleared by law enforcement. This is sometimes called "staging for PD."

D. Accident Scenes

1. Extrication situations. Federal law requires EMS workers wear an approved highly reflective traffic safety vest when working on roadways, around traffic, or at an accident scene.

E. Additional Hazards Requiring Specially Trained Responders

1. Downed power lines, fire situations, etc.

2. Terrorism incidents involving chemical, biological, radiological, nuclear, or explosive hazards

3. High-angle rescue, swift-water rescue, confined space rescue, etc.

V. LIFTING AND MOVING

A. Patient Safety. Use extreme caution when lifting and moving patients. This is a high-risk activity for both patients and providers.

B. Safe Lifting Techniques

1. Power lift. Keep object close to the body. Use the legs to lift, not the back (legs bent, back straight). Use a power grip with palms up and all fingers wrapped around the object.

2. Position the stretcher to reduce the height of the lift.

3. Preplan the lift to reduce distance and avoid problems.

4. Get enough help.

C. Emergency Moves. These are used when the scene is dangerous and the patient must be moved before providing patient care. Types of emergency moves include the armpit-forearm drag, shirt drag, and blanket drag.

D. Urgent Move

1. Used when the patient has potentially life-threatening injuries or illness and must be moved quickly for evaluation and transport.

2. Rapid extrication: an urgent move used for patients in a motor vehicle; it requires multiple rescuers and a long backboard. The patient is rotated onto a backboard with manual cervical spine precautions and removed from the vehicle.

E. Non-Urgent Moves

1. Used when there are no hazards and no life-threatening conditions apparent.

2. Types of non-urgent moves include direct ground lift, extremity lift, direct carry method, and draw sheet method.

F. Log Roll Technique

1. Commonly used to place a patient on a backboard or assess the posterior.

2. Can be done while maintaining manual cervical spine precautions.

3. Should have at least three trained personnel. The person controlling manual cervical spine protection should direct the log roll.

G. Equipment for Patient Movement

1. Wheeled stretcher: a stretcher that secures in the ambulance for transport and is usually the safest way to move a patient. Most models can accommodate at least 300 pounds. Newer models have an automated lift system to further reduce the risk of injury.

2. Portable stretcher: a lightweight and compact stretcher that allows more accessibility than wheeled stretchers.

3. Stair chair: excellent for staircases, small elevators, etc. A stair chair, however, does not allow for manual cervical spine protection, CPR, or artificial ventilation.

4. Backboard: used primarily for cervical spine immobilization, a backboard is lightweight and allows for CPR and artificial ventilation. Requires a four-person lift.

5. Scoop stretcher: most scoop stretchers separate into two long pieces (left and right, not top to bottom). Allows for easy positioning with minimal patient movement. Good for reducing patient discomfort during movement compared to other techniques.

6. Neonatal isolette: designed to keep neonatal patients warm during transport; requires specialized training to operate.

7. Patient packaging for air medical transport

    i. If there is a hazardous material exposure, patient must be decontaminated before being loaded onto the aircraft.

    ii. Notify air medical crew ASAP of any special circumstances, such as a large patient, cardiac arrest patient, traction splint applied, combative patient, or unstable airway.

    iii. Secure all loose equipment, blankets, etc., before approaching a running aircraft.

    iv. Never approach the aircraft without pilot or air medical crew authorization.

    v. Never approach a rotor wing aircraft from the rear. Never back up.

H. Special Considerations

1. Bariatric (obese) patients

    i. Obese patients pose additional challenges and risks to providers during lifting and movement. Know what your equipment (stretcher, backboard, etc.) is capable of holding. Request additional assistance.

    ii. Some EMS systems have special bariatric ambulances with specialized equipment, automated lifting systems, and wider stretchers capable of a greater weight capacity.

2. Skeletal abnormalities. Patients with unusual curvature of the spine, such as kyphosis or lordosis, may not be capable of lying supine without special padding.

3. Pregnant patients. Patients in the later stages of pregnancy should not be placed supine due to the risk of supine hypotensive syndrome. Place the pregnant patient on her left side. If patient has potential cervical spine trauma, tilt backboard to the left about 20 degrees.

VI. MEDICAL RESTRAINT

A. Laws and protocols vary widely. In general, patients may be forcibly restrained if they pose a significant, immediate threat to you, your partner, or others.

   1. Restraining a patient against his will is a last resort.

   2. Anticipate and plan. Request law enforcement assistance. Know your local protocols. Contact medical direction when possible.

   3. Guidelines for restraining a patient

      i. Get additional help whenever possible; at least four people is recommended.

      ii. Use the minimum amount of force necessary to protect yourself, the patient, and others.

      iii. Secure patient supine, with a backboard if available. Do *not* secure the patient in the prone position.

      iv. Use soft, padded restraints. Avoid handcuffs, flex-cuffs, etc.

      v. Monitor the patient's level of consciousness, airway, and distal circulation (below point of restraints) continuously.

      vi. Thoroughly document the reason for restraining the patient, the method of restraint, the duration of restraint, and frequent reassessment of the patient while restrained.

      vii. Do *not* ever restrain a patient in the prone position, hogtie a patient, or leave a restrained patient unsupervised.

B. Use of Force Doctrine. The EMT must act reasonably to prevent harm to a patient being forcibly restrained. The use of force must be protective, *not* punitive.

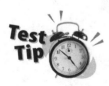

Security for the NREMT exam is rigorous. The questions on the exam come from an extensive unpublished database. Candidates cannot view the questions in advance. The only way to pass the test is to possess the necessary knowledge and good test-taking skills. This book will help you with both!

PRACTICE QUESTIONS

1. You are called to a business for a patient with dizziness, headache, and nausea. As you enter the business, you detect a strong odor and your eyes begin to water. You should immediately

   A. leave the area and call for additional resources.

   B. attempt to locate the caller and remove him.

   C. apply a mask and safety goggles before continuing.

   D. determine the cause of the odor and notify your dispatcher.

2. Which of the following statements regarding stress is correct?

   A. EMTs can avoid stress by eating healthy and exercising.

   B. Stress will eventually cause most EMTs to leave the profession.

   C. Stress is an inevitable consequence of the profession.

   D. Acute stress develops slowly due to repeat exposure to certain events.

3. Which of the following is a formalized process to help emergency workers deal with stress?

   A. paid time off

   B. modified duty assignment

   C. critical incident stress management

   D. EMS stress management exercises

4. Which of the following provides the best protection from exposure to an airborne disease?

   A. HEPA mask

   B. simple mask

   C. long-sleeve gown

   D. mask with splash guard

5. Which of the following moves is used when the scene is dangerous and the patient must be moved before providing care?

   A. urgent move

   B. emergency move

   C. non-urgent move

   D. critical move

ANSWERS:

1. **A.**

   This is a scene safety question. Expect to be asked several versions of this question on your NREMT exam. Your safety is *always* the first priority.

2. **C.**

   Stress is inevitable in EMS, but there are ways to manage it. Acute stress is an immediate physiological and psychological reaction to a specific event.

3. **C.**

   CISM (critical incident stress management) is a formalized process to help emergency workers deal with stress. Paid time off and modified duty assignments are not formally recognized stress management techniques. EMS stress management exercises? We made up that one!

4. **A.**

   A HEPA mask or N95 mask should be worn if you suspect the patient has an airborne disease. The other options provide little or no protection from airborne diseases.

5. **B.**

   Emergency moves are used when the scene is dangerous and the patient must be moved immediately. Urgent moves are used when the patient has life-threatening injuries. There is no such thing as a "critical" move.

Medical, Legal, and Ethical Issues, and EMS Research

I. MEDICAL/LEGAL CONSIDERATIONS

A. Medical Direction

1. EMS providers operate under the license of their physician medical director(s).

2. It is essential for EMTs to know the standing orders, guidelines, and protocols for their state, agency, and medical director.

3. Always contact the appropriate medical direction authority if you are unsure how to manage a patient.

B. Scope of Practice

1. Scope of practice outlines the actions a provider is legally allowed to perform based on his or her license or certification level.

2. Scope of practice is tied to the licensure or certification, not the individual's knowledge or experience. For example, former military medics cannot exceed the scope of practice for their civilian certification level despite the likelihood they are capable of doing so.

3. Each state determines the scope of practice for its EMS providers. The National EMS Education Standards (NEMSES) attempts to better align scope of practice throughout the United States.

C. Standard of Care

1. Standard of care is the degree of care a reasonable person with similar training would provide in a similar situation.

2. Standard of care applies the "reasonable person test": Would a reasonable person with the same training do the same thing in the same situation?

3. Standard of care requires EMTs to competently perform the indicated assessment and treatment within their scope of practice.

4. Sources that help establish standard of care

   i. National EMS Education Standards

   ii. State protocols and guidelines

   iii. Medical direction

   iv. EMS agency's policies and procedures

   v. Reputable textbooks

   vi. Care considered acceptable by similarly trained providers in the same community

D. Consent

   1. Informed consent is required from all patients who are alert and competent.

      i. Patient must be informed of your care plan and associated risks of accepting or refusing care and transport.

      ii. Patient must be informed of, and understand, all information that would impact a reasonable person's decision to accept or refuse care and transport.

   2. Expressed consent also requires that the patient be alert and competent to give expressed consent. Expressed consent can be given verbally or nonverbally.

      i. Expressed consent is similar to informed consent, but not usually as in-depth as informed consent.

      ii. Expressed consent is often used to obtain consent for more basic assessments or procedures.

   3. Implied consent allows assumption of consent for emergency care from an unresponsive or incompetent patient.

      i. Patients might be incompetent for many reasons, such as alcohol, drugs, head injury, hypoxia, hypoglycemia, or mental incompetency.

      ii. Implied consent can be used to treat a patient who initially refused care but later loses consciousness or becomes otherwise incapacitated.

   4. Minor consent. Minors are not competent to accept or refuse care.

      i.   Consent is required from a parent or legal guardian. Implied consent can be used when unable to reach a parent or guardian and treatment is needed.

      ii.   Minor consent is not required for emancipated minors. Criteria for emancipation varies but usually includes minors who are married or pregnant, already a parent, a member of the armed forces, financially independent, or emancipated by the courts.

  5. Involuntary consent is used for mentally incompetent adults or those in custody of law enforcement. Consent must be obtained from the entity with the appropriate legal authority.

E. Advance Directives

  1. Advance directives are written instructions, signed by the patient, specifying the patient's wishes regarding treatment and resuscitative efforts. There are several types of advance directives:

      i.   Do Not Resuscitate (DNR). DNRs are specific to resuscitation efforts and do not affect treatment prior to the patient entering cardiac arrest.

      ii.   Living will. Living wills are broader than DNRs. They address health-care wishes prior to entering cardiac arrest. This may include use of advanced airways, ventilators, feeding tubes, etc.

  2. Requirements for a legally recognized advance directive vary by state. Consult local protocols.

F. EMT Liability

  1. Good Samaritan laws. Good Samaritan laws are designed to protect someone who renders care as long as he or she is not being compensated and gross negligence is not committed.

      i.   Each state has some form of Good Samaritan law. Some protect health-care providers, but some do not.

      ii.   Some states extend their Good Samaritan law to publicly employed EMS providers but not to those in the private sector.

  2. Criminal liability

      i.   Criminal law involves a government entity taking legal action against a person. Criminal complaints include the following:

        ➤ Assault. A person can be guilty of assault even if another person only perceived that they intended to inflict harm. Physical contact is not required to be guilty of assault.

        ➤ Battery. Battery is physically touching another person without their consent.

    ii. If an EMT is found to be criminally liable, he or she may face imprisonment and loss of certification.

3. Civil liability

    i. In civil law, an individual (plaintiff) sues an EMT (defendant) for a wrongful act involving injury or damage.

    ii. A civil suit may also involve multiple EMS providers, employers, supervisors, training programs, and medical directors.

    iii. In a civil suit, the plaintiff(s) seeks monetary compensation from the defendant(s).

4. Negligence is the most common reason EMS providers are sued civilly.

    i. The plaintiff has the burden of proof, not the EMT.

    ii. With negligence, the EMS provider is accused of unintentional harm to the plaintiff.

    iii. The plaintiff must prove all four of the following:

        ➤ Duty to act. The EMT had an obligation to respond and provide care.

        ➤ Breach of duty. The EMT failed to assess, treat, or transport patient according to the standard of care.

        ➤ Damage. The plaintiff experienced damage or injury recognized by the legal system as worthy of compensation.

        ➤ Causation (also called "proximate cause"). The injury to the plaintiff was, at least in part, directly due to the EMT's breech of duty.

    iv. Gross negligence

        ➤ Gross negligence exceeds simple negligence. Gross negligence involves an indifference to, and violation of, a legal responsibility.

➤ Reckless patient care that is clearly dangerous to the patient is grossly negligent.

➤ Gross negligence can result in civil and/or criminal charges.

5. Abandonment

   i.   Once care is initiated, EMS providers cannot terminate care without the patient's consent. Some patient encounters may also require direct contact with medical direction prior to terminating care. Most EMS agencies have written protocols for terminating care without transporting the patient to a higher level of care.

  ii.   Abandonment is the termination of care without transferring the patient to an equal or higher medical authority. Transfer of care must include a verbal report to an equal or higher medical authority. Most EMS systems allow EMTs to accept care from a paramedic or advanced EMT for transport if an advanced-level assessment or advanced care is not needed.

6. False imprisonment. You may be guilty of false imprisonment if you transport a competent patient without consent.

7. Hospital destination

   i.   The choice of hospital destination when transporting a patient is a growing source of litigation against EMS providers. Destination factors include

➤ the patient's request or medical direction

➤ the closest appropriate facility or specialty facility

➤ written protocols or triage guidelines

➤ hospital diversion or bypass

  ii.   Follow local and federal guidelines.

 iii.   A patient's ability to pay should *not* factor into where a patient is transported.

 iv.   When in doubt, consult medical direction.

  v.   Thoroughly document why the destination was chosen. This is especially true if you bypass a closer hospital capable of managing your patient.

8. Patient refusals. Competent patients may refuse treatment regardless of the severity of their condition.

i. Refusals present high liability risk for EMS providers.

ii. Negligence or abandonment can be much easier to prove if the patient is not transported.

iii. Consider requesting advanced life support personnel or contacting medical direction per local protocols.

iv. Typically, competency requires awareness of at least four things:

> ➤ Person. The patient knows his or her name.

> ➤ Place. The patient knows where he or she is.

> ➤ Time. The patient is aware of the date and time.

> ➤ Event. The patient is aware of his or her present circumstances.

> ➤ Additional considerations affecting competency:

>> — Is the patient of legal age?

>> — Does the patient appear impaired by drugs or alcohol?

>> — Does the patient appear mentally impaired by significant illness or injury?

>> — Are there any communication barriers, such as language or ability to hear?

v. During a refusal, the patient must be fully informed of the treatment recommended and the possible consequences of refusing treatment.

vi. Reducing liability on a patient refusal

> ➤ Ensure the patient is absolutely competent.

> ➤ The EMT's best protection from liability is to provide excellent care and convince the patient to accept transport.

> ➤ The second best way for an EMT to protect him- or herself is to ensure the patient is fully informed, contact medical direction, and document extremely well.

vii. Documentation. The patient is rarely, if ever, fully informed the first time he or she conveys the intent to refuse treatment. Documentation should reflect both the initial refusal and the second refusal after being fully informed.

➤ Document the patient's awareness of person, place, time, and event.

➤ Document all the information you provided to the patient so he or she can make an informed decision.

➤ Document any advice given to the patient.

➤ Document that the patient is aware he can always change his mind and call EMS again at any time.

➤ Accurately document all times, including patient contact and departure times, vitals, any treatment, etc.

➤ Document at least two sets of vitals.

➤ Accurately document the assessments and treatments that were performed, including response to treatment.

➤ Document consultation with medical direction and any orders received.

➤ Obtain the patient's signature and the signature of a witness (not another EMS provider).

➤ If your agency has an approved refusal of care form, use it.

G. Patient Confidentiality

1. In most cases, EMS providers cannot release confidential patient information without written consent.

2. EMTs can release confidential patient information without consent when

   i.   the information is necessary for continuity of care

   ii. the information is necessary to facilitate billing for services

   iii. the EMT has received a valid subpoena

   iv. reporting possible crimes, abuse, assault, neglect, certain injuries, or communicable diseases

3. Health Insurance Portability and Accountability Act (HIPAA)

   i.   HIPAA is a federal law established in 1996 and has had a huge impact on health care. HIPAA improved privacy protection of patient health care records.

   ii. HIPAA gives patients greater control over how health care records are used and transferred.

      iii. EMS agencies are mandated to provide HIPAA training to all employees who have any contact with patients or patient records.

      iv. EMS providers must provide patients with privacy practices and obtain signature of receipt.

H. Consolidated Omnibus Budget Reconciliation Act (COBRA) and Emergency Medical Treatment and Active Labor Act (EMTALA)

  1. COBRA and EMTALA include federal regulations guaranteeing public access to emergency care.

  2. COBRA and EMTALA are also intended to stop the inappropriate transfer of patients, known as a patient "dump."

I. Interfacility Transports

  1. Obtain a patient report from the transferring facility before departing.

  2. Confirm the exact destination location, including department or admitting physician.

  3. Make sure the patient's condition does not exceed scope of practice.

  4. Obtain consent from the patient or guardian.

J. Death Determination

  1. Local protocols vary on whether EMS personnel have the authority to declare death. Consult local protocol. When in doubt, contact medical direction.

  2. Signs of death can be presumptive or definitive. Presumptive signs typically indicate the need to begin resuscitation and include unresponsiveness, pulselessness, and apnea. Definitive or obvious signs of death typically indicate that resuscitation should *not* be initiated. The following are typically considered definitive signs of death:

      i. Decomposition: physical decay of the body's components

      ii. Rigor mortis: stiffening of the body after death

      iii. Dependent lividity: the settling of blood within the body

    iv. Decapitation: the patient's head is no longer attached to the body

K. Notification of Authorities. Law enforcement or the medical examiner must typically be notified for situations including:

1. any scene where the patient is dead on arrival

2. suicide attempts

3. assault or sexual assault

4. child abuse or elder abuse

5. suspected crime scene

6. childbirth

L. Crime Scenes

1. Ensure scene safety.

2. Provide patient care as needed.

3. Avoid any unnecessary disturbance of scene.

4. Remember and note the position of patient(s).

5. Remember and report everything you touched at the scene.

6. Cut around (not through) holes in clothing when exposing the patient.

7. Note anything or anyone suspicious on or near the scene.

8. Discourage sexual assault patients from changing clothes or showering.

9. Try to get a same-sex provider to assist with sexual assault patients.

10. Leave once you are no longer needed on the scene.

M. Organ Donors

1. Proof of intent to donate organs is usually obtained through a signed donor card or driver's license.

2. Treat the patient as you normally would.

3. Notify medical direction and receiving personnel at the hospital.

II. **PROFESSIONAL ETHICS FOR EMS PROVIDERS**

A. Ethics are the moral principles that guide a person or group, in this case, the EMS profession. "Bioethics" is specific to ethical issues related to health care.

B. All EMS calls present some sort of ethical issue.

C. The EMT Oath and Code of Ethics can be found on the National Association of EMTs website at *www.naemt.org/About_EMS/emtoath.aspx*.

D. Personal morals, professional ethics, and the law. An EMT's moral, ethical, and legal obligations do not usually conflict with one another. For example, all three require that an EMT document what he or she did, not what should have been done.

1. Sometimes, conflicts do arise. When in doubt,

   i. consider what is best for the patient

   ii. know the law and your protocols

   iii. get help from your partner, your supervisor, ALS personnel, or medical direction, etc.

2. Potential ethical conflicts

   i. Triage at mass casualty incidents

   ii. Coercive refusals

   iii. Futile resuscitation attempts

III. **EMS RESEARCH**

A. Traditionally, EMS protocols have been based on practices and guidelines handed down by higher medical authorities.

1. In many cases, these practices were not based on research or were based on in-hospital practices.

2. In some cases, these practices did not improve patient outcomes.

3. In a few cases, these practices proved harmful to patients.

B. Evidence-based Medicine

1. The EMS profession must, and has begun to, take responsibility for basing decisions on research.

2. The amount of prehospital-based research is growing.

3. For additional information on EMS research, visit the Prehospital Care Research Forum at *www.cpc.mednet.ucla.edu/pcrf*.

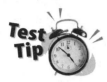

The certification exam is a computer-adaptive test. This means no two people will take the same exact test. The test is constantly adapting to the test taker's previous responses.

The question's topic and level of difficulty, and the test taker's response all affect what comes next. Once you submit your answer, you cannot go back and change your response.

PRACTICE QUESTIONS

1. Which of the following terms refers to the actions an EMS provider is legally allowed to perform based on his or her license or certification level?

   A. duty to act

   B. standard of care

   C. scope of practice

   D. doctrine of certification

2. Which of the following terms refers to the degree of care a reasonable person with similar training should provide in a similar situation?

   A. standard of care

   B. scope of practice

   C. standardized curriculum

   D. EMS expectation clause

3. Which of the following are specific to resuscitation efforts and do not affect treatment prior to the patient entering cardiac arrest?

   A. living will

   B. advance directive

   C. DNR order

   D. medical power of attorney

4. During a negligence lawsuit, it is shown that the injury to the plaintiff was, at least in part, directly due to the EMT's action or inaction. Which component of negligence is the EMT guilty of?

   A. proximate cause

   B. duty to act

   C. breech of duty

   D. gross incompetence

5. Which of the following is a definitive sign of death?

   A. decapitation

   B. pulselessness

   C. apnea

   D. unresponsiveness

ANSWERS

1. C.

   This question defines the scope of practice. It is important to understand the difference between the scope of practice and the standard of care. "Duty to act" is one of the four components of negligence. There is no "doctrine of certification."

2. A.

   This question defines the standard of care. There is no "EMS expectation clause."

3. **C.**

   DNR orders only apply to patients once they enter cardiac arrest. This is not always true of living wills or advance directives.

4. **A.**

   This question defines the proximate cause or "causation" component of negligence. Gross negligence involves an indifference to, and violation of, a legal responsibility.

5. **A.**

   Decapitation is a definitive sign of death. The other answer choices are presumptive signs of death. It is important to know the difference between presumptive and definitive signs of death. Definitive signs include decapitation, dependent lividity, decomposition, and rigor mortis.

Communications

I. INTRODUCTION TO COMMUNICATIONS

A. EMS communications typically relate to mobile-based communications with dispatch, medical direction, other emergency service workers, etc.

B. Therapeutic communications typically refers to your interaction with the patient and ability to obtain clinical information.

C. Interpersonal communications is the ability to send and receive information between at least two people.

II. EMS COMMUNICATIONS

A. Portable radios: hand-held transmitter/receiver with a very limited range, unless used with a repeater.

B. Mobile radios: vehicle-mounted transmitters and receivers. These have a greater range than portable radios, but distance is still limited unless used with a repeater.

C. Repeater: a type of base station that receives low-power transmissions from portable or mobile radios and rebroadcasts at higher power to improve range.

D. Base station: a transmitter/receiver in a fixed location that is in contact with all other components in the radio system.

E. Mobile Data Computers (MDCs)

1. Relay digital information instead of voice transmissions

    2. Can display the address of the call and routing information

    3. Allow digital communication with dispatch and other responding units

    4. Reduce the volume of routine radio traffic

F. Cellular Phones

    1. Cellular phones are quickly replacing radio communication with medical direction.

    2. Advantages include easy, clear, inexpensive means of communication.

    3. Disadvantages include potential unreliability communication during peak demand or a mass casualty incident.

G. Federal Communications Commission (FCC). The FCC regulates all radio operations in the United States and has allocated specific frequencies for EMS use only.

H. Guidelines for Radio Communication

    1. Communication with dispatch

        i.   Confirm receipt of dispatch.

        ii. Notify dispatch when en route to the call, on scene, en route to the hospital, and at the hospital.

    2. Do

        i.   make sure you are on the correct frequency.

        ii. ensure there is no other radio traffic before transmitting.

        iii. depress the transmit button and wait one second before speaking.

        iv. identify who you are talking to first, then who you are. For example, "Dispatch, this is medic 1."

        v. use clear text, not radio codes unless approved locally.

        vi. use "affirmative" or "negative," not "yes" or "no."

        vii. use "copy" to confirm receipt of a transmission.

        viii. always "echo" orders from medical direction to confirm accuracy.

3. Do *not*

    i.   use unnecessary verbiage, such as "please" or "thank you."

    ii. relay protected information such as the patient's name.

I. Communicating with Medical Direction

1. Communication with medical direction often involves relaying a lot of information clearly in a short period of time.

2. Details matter, and mutual understanding is critical.

3. Strong verbal communication skills are needed. Body language won't help over the phone or radio.

4. Provide objective information, not subjective opinions.

5. Each call and patient is different; however, patient information should always be relayed from high priority to low priority.

6. Sample format for relaying patient information

    i.   Unit designation, certification level, destination, and estimated time of arrival (ETA)

    ii. Patient's age, sex, chief complaint

    iii. Patient's level of consciousness

    iv. History of present illness or mechanism of injury

    v.   Any associated symptoms or pertinent negatives

    vi. Patient's vitals

    vii. Patient's physical exam

    viii. Patient's history, medications, allergies

    ix. Treatment provided and response to treatment

    x.   Any requests for additional interventions

    xi. Echo any orders provided by medical direction

J. Transfer of Care

1. Verbal report. Transfer of care must include a verbal report to an equal or higher medical authority. Provide all relevant information similar to radio report, including any changes since the radio report.

2. A written copy of the patient care report must also be provided.

3. The same principles apply to the transfer of patients between prehospital providers.

 III. **INTERPERSONAL COMMUNICATION**

A. Sending and Receiving Verbal Communications

1. The message sender "encodes" the message, and the receiver "decodes" the message.

2. While communicating, senders and receivers can trade rolls often.

3. Radio communication can limit transfer of rolls if only one person can transmit or receive at once.

4. What the sender meant to convey (imply) may not be what the receiver interpreted (inferred).

B. Factors That Influence Communication

1. Nonverbal cues, such as body language, have a huge impact on communication. These can be lost during radio or cellular communication.

2. Your attitude and tone have a significant impact on effectiveness of communication.

C. Establishing Rapport with the Patient

1. You should introduce yourself.

2. Ask for the patient's name and use it.

3. Make eye contact with the patient.

4. Be honest.

5. Use age-appropriate techniques.

6. Be aware of special needs, such as those for hearing-impaired patients.

7. Respect cultural differences.

D. When communicating with the patient, you should *not*

1. make promises you can't deliver

2. lie to or mislead the patient

3. give advice beyond your scope of practice

4. use biased or judgmental questions such as "Why . . . "

5. interrupt the patient

6. use confrontational techniques or overexert your authority

7. overuse medical terms or professional lingo

E. Challenging Communication Situations

1. Patients with special challenges (hearing or visually impaired patients; patients who are developmentally disabled; patients who speak a different language)

2. Patients under the influence of drugs or alcohol

3. Pediatric patients

IV. THERAPEUTIC COMMUNICATION

A. Compassion. Clearly communicate you are concerned for the patient's well-being. Show empathy (the ability to see things from the patient's perspective).

B. Competence. The EMT must communicate competence, both verbally and nonverbally.

C. Confidence. Communicate that you are a professional and you know what needs to be done.

D. Conscience. Communicate, through your actions, that you are following the ethical standards established by your profession.

E. Commitment. Communicate to everyone you are committed to whatever is best for the patient.

F. Questioning Patients

1. Listen! Listening to your patients' responses is the most important part of being an EMT.

2. Ask patients the most important questions first.

3. Open-ended questions are often preferred. For example, "Can you tell us what's wrong today?" instead of "Are you having chest pain?"

4. Use closed questions when you need specific information or the patient is unable to provide longer answers.

5. Avoid judgmental or biased questions.

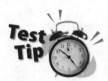

You don't need to achieve a specific score on the exam. You are being evaluated for "entry-level competency." The test is extremely accurate at assessing competency. There is no substitute for being thoroughly prepared. You can do it!

PRACTICE QUESTIONS

1. What federal agency regulates all radio operations in the United States?

   A. Federal Trade Commission

   B. Department of Transportation

   C. National Registry of EMTs

   D. Federal Communications Commission

2. Which of the following statements regarding EMS radio communications is correct?

   A. Begin and end radio transmissions with "please" and "thank you."

   B. Use the 10 codes approved by the NREMT.

   C. Use clear text, not radio codes, for EMS communications.

   D. State "over and out" and the end of each radio transmission.

3. Which of the following is an example of an objective observation?

   A. "The patient has slurred speech and an unsteady gait."

   B. "The patient is high on something."

   C. "The patient is obviously intoxicated."

   D. "The patient is under the influence of alcohol or drugs."

4. Your medical direction has just ordered administration of a medication for your patient. You should immediately

   A. administer the medication as directed.

   B. check with one additional physician to confirm the order is correct.

   C. repeat the order back to ensure you have understood it correctly.

   D. ask the physician to verbally acknowledge that you are allowed to give the medication.

5. Which of the following statements regarding the transfer of care report is correct?

   A. Transfer of care must always be to the accepting physician.

   B. Transfer of care must include a verbal report to an equal or higher medical authority.

   C. Transfer of care is not allowed until you complete your documentation form.

   D. Transfer of care can be made to anyone as long as the patient agrees.

ANSWERS

1. **D.**

   The FCC regulates all radio communications in the U.S. The NREMT is not a federal agency.

2. **C.**

   Use clear text, not radio codes, unless approved locally.

3. **A.**

   The correct answer demonstrates an objective observation. The other answer choices are subjective opinions.

4. **C.**

   Always repeat the order back (known as echoing) to ensure you heard it correctly. This should be done before the medication is administered.

5. **B.**

   Transfer of care must be made to an equal or higher medical authority. A copy of the PCR must be provided, but it does *not* delay transfer of care.

Documentation

I. PURPOSES OF THE PATIENT CARE REPORT (PCR)

A. Continuation of Care. Your PCR provides important information to those that will continue patient care after your work is done.

B. Legal Document

1. Your PCR becomes part of the patient's permanent medical record.

2. Typically, the person who wrote the PCR will be the person subpoenaed to give a deposition or testify in court.

3. *Documentation rule No. 1:* If you did it, write it down. If you didn't do it, don't write that you did.

4. *Documentation rule No. 2:* It is much better to document well than to explain later why you didn't.

C. Billing. Your PCR may be used to correctly bill the patient or insurance company for services provided.

D. Research and Continuous Quality Improvement. Data from your PCR will likely contribute to numerous research and CQI projects.

II. MINIMUM DATA SET

A. The minimum data set identifies the information that should be included on every PCR.

B. Times

1. The following times should be recorded:

   i. Dispatch time

        ii.   Time en route to call

        iii. Time on scene

        iv. Patient contact time

        v.   Time en route to hospital

        vi. Arrival time at hospital

        vii. Time transfer of care was completed

  2. Importance of time on the PCR

        i.   Accurate times are critical. The clock on the electrocardiogram (ECG) monitor and watches or phones of all EMS providers should be synchronized with the clock in the dispatch center.

        ii. Inaccurate times are an easy target for litigators. It calls into question the validity of your entire PCR.

        iii. *Documentation rule No. 3:* If your times are proven inaccurate, you may be in for a miserable deposition or courtroom experience.

C. Patient Information

  1. The patient's age, sex, and chief complaint

  2. The patient's level of consciousness

  3. Minimum of two sets of vital signs

  4. All assessments completed on the patient

  5. All treatments provided and response to treatment

D. Administrative Information

  1. The address of call

  2. Date of call

  3. Your unit designation

  4. The name or identifying number and certification level of all EMS providers on the call

E. Narrative. This is where the EMT "paints the picture" of what happened. Usually, this is the first place readers will go to begin understanding the call.

DOCUMENTATION GUIDELINES

A. **F.A.C.T.** Documentation

1. **F**actual. The PCR should be fact-based, not opinion-based.

2. **A**ccurate. The PCR should be as accurate as possible. Never falsify a PCR.

3. **C**omplete. The PCR should be complete unless special circumstances dictate otherwise, such as a mass casualty incident. Complete does *not* mean you document things that were not actually done. If an area of the PCR was not completed, document "not completed" and document why.

4. **T**imely. The PCR should be completed as soon as possible after transfer of care. It is a good idea to document the time the PCR was completed.

B. *Documentation rule No. 4:* Document objectively, not subjectively.

1. Objective documentation is based on facts, findings, or observations that are highly difficult to dispute. Objective documentation is not about being "right."

2. Subjective documentation is based on opinions or perceptions and can be easily disputed. Subjective documentation is about being "right" about your opinion. Subjective information from the patient, however, is acceptable and should generally be documented in quotations.

3. Examples of objective and subjective documentation

   i. Objective: "Patient with pain and deformity to elbow." Subjective: "Patient with dislocated elbow."

   ii. Objective: "Patient states he drank two beers this evening." Subjective: "Patient intoxicated."

C. Associated Symptoms and Pertinent Negatives. It is important to document associated symptoms and relevant pertinent negatives.

1. Associated symptoms: patient complaints in addition to the chief complaint. For example, the chief complaint is chest pain, but the patient also complains of mild difficulty breathing.

2. Pertinent negatives: signs or symptoms you have reason to suspect but the patient denies having. For example, the patient experienced trauma but denies neck pain.

D. Abbreviations

1. Most agencies have a list of approved abbreviations. Abbreviations not on your agency's approved list should *not* be used.

2. *Documentation rule No. 5:* Spelling counts! If your PCR has a spell-check feature, use it. If your PCR is handwritten and you make more than two spelling errors, start over if time permits.

E. Errors and Falsifications

1. Draw a single line through the middle of any mistake(s). Initial the mistake and make the correction. Never scribble out a mistake so it cannot be read.

2. Intentional falsification of a PCR jeopardizes patient care. It is also grounds for termination, revocation of certification, and possible legal action. Components commonly falsified on a PCR include vital signs, assessment and treatment areas, and times.

3. Errors of omission. An error of omission means something that should have been included was left out of the PCR.

4. Errors of commission. Something incorrect was included on the PCR.

 IV. PATIENT REFUSALS

A. Thoroughly document the patient's competency.

B. Document your assessment. If unable to complete an appropriate assessment, document why.

C. Document any treatment provided and response to treatment. Document any attempted treatment the patient refused.

D. Document at least two sets of vitals. If two sets are not provided, document why.

E. Document your recommendation the patient be treated and transported.

F. Document your discussion about the possible risks of refusing treatment.

G. Document that the patient understood the information provided and made an informed decision to refuse treatment.

H. Document your discussion with medical direction.

I. Document your recommendation the patient call again if he changes his mind or gets worse.

J. Obtain the patient's signature on the refusal form.

K. Obtain a signature from a witness, but not a fellow EMS provider.

V. ELECTRONIC PCRS (E-PCR)

A. Pros of e-PCRs

1. Improvement of data storage and retrieval

2. Improved ability to use PCR information for CQI and research

3. This is now the standard for the EMS profession.

B. Cons of e-PCR

1. Some find e-PCRs more difficult to "paint" a clear picture of the call.

2. It is difficult to design software that is easy for users to adjust to and detailed enough to capture all necessary information.

3. Transfer of e-PCRs during transfer of care can be challenging.

VI. SPECIAL REPORTING SITUATIONS

A. In most EMS systems, certain circumstances require special documentation or notification in addition to or in place of the PCR.

1. Mass casualty incidents. During a mass casualty incident (MCI), the triage tag may be the only documentation of patient care.

2. Suspected cases of abuse or criminal activity

3. Animal bites

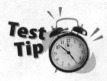

Everyone taking the test will feel pushed to the limits of his or her abilities. The software driving the test ensures you will get questions challenging for you. It's important to stay focused, read carefully, and not get discouraged during the test.

PRACTICE QUESTIONS

1. Which of the following suggestions should you follow regarding patient care reports?

    A. Always keep a copy of the PCR for your own records.

    B. If you didn't do it, don't write that you did.

    C. Have the patient review the PCR once it is complete.

    D. Leave your name off the PCR if you have concerns about the call.

2. The minimum data set on a PCR includes

    A. dispatch times.

    B. patient diagnosis.

    C. insurance information.

    D. the medical director's name.

3. Your PCR has a section that allows you to free text a description of the call. This is known as the

    A. dispatch section.

    B. treatment section.

    C. physical exam section.

    D. narrative section.

4. Your patient is complaining of knee pain following a fall from a bicycle. You ask the patient if he has any neck pain and he states he does not. In this case, neck pain would be considered

   A. a pertinent negative.

   B. an associated symptom.

   C. multi-system trauma.

   D. an irrelevant question.

5. What abbreviations should you use on your PCR?

   A. any abbreviation you like, as long as you are consistent

   B. any abbreviation a senior EMT or paramedic uses

   C. only abbreviations approved by your agency and medical director

   D. only abbreviations approved by the NREMT

ANSWERS

1. **B.**

   All other answer choices are completely inappropriate.

2. **A.**

   The minimum data set includes information that should be on every PCR, such as dispatch times.

3. **D.**

   The narrative section allows you to describe the call in your own words.

4. **A.**

   The question is relevant and important to ask. Since it's not present, it would be considered a pertinent negative. If the patient answered "yes," then neck pain would be considered an associated symptom.

5. **C.**

   You should only use abbreviations approved by your agency and medical director. The NREMT does not approve medical abbreviations.

Anatomy and Physiology/ Medical Terminology

I. KEY TOPICS

A. Anatomy: the study of the body's structure

B. Physiology: the study of the body's function

C. Pathophysiology: the study of disease

II. HOMEOSTASIS

A. Homeostasis is a state of balance or equilibrium within the body.

B. Every cell, tissue, organ, and system in the human body functions to maintain homeostasis.

C. The human body's homeostatic range is quite narrow.

III. TOPOGRAPHIC ANATOMY

A. There are numerous terms used to reference locations on the outer surface of the body. All terms are based on the body being in the "anatomical position."

B. Anatomical position: the body is in the standing position, arms at the sides, with palms forward (thumbs on the outside).

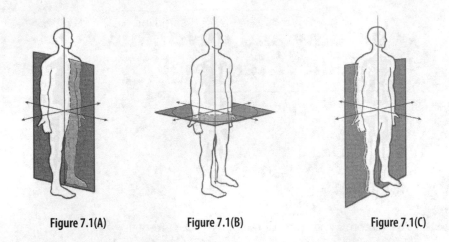

| Figure 7.1(A) | Figure 7.1(B) | Figure 7.1(C) |

C. Planes of the Body

1. The midline divides the body into left and right. (A)

2. The transverse plane divides the body into top and bottom at the level of the umbilicus (belly button). (B)

3. The frontal plane (imaginary line) divides the body into anterior and posterior. (C)

D. Paired Directional Terms

1. Anterior or ventral (front) and posterior or dorsal (back)

2. Superior (top) and inferior (bottom)

3. Proximal (closer to point of attachment) and distal (farther from point of attachment)

4. Medial (close to midline) and lateral (far from midline)

E. Terms of Movement

1. Abduction: movement away from midline

   i. Example: Assume the anatomical position; lift your arms straight up at your sides (not in front of you). This is abduction.

2. Adduction: movement toward the midline

    i.   Example: With your arms straight out at your sides, move them down to anatomical position. This is adduction.

3. Extension: straightening the joint (increasing the angle of the joint).

    i.   Example: Bend your arm so there is a 90-degree angle between your forearm and upper arm (flexed bicep position). Extend the arm so both portions of the arm form a straight line. This is extension.

4. Flexion: bending the joint (decreasing the angle of the joint).

    i.   Example: Stand in the anatomical position. Leave your upper leg in position, bend at the knee, and lift the lower leg up behind you. This is flexion.

F. Body Positions

1. Supine: lying on you back, face up

2. Prone: lying on your stomach, face down

3. Fowler position: seated with head elevated

4. Recovery position: lying on the left or right side

NOTE: The use of Trendelenburg or "shock position" is no longer recommended.

G. Abdominal Quadrants. The four abdominal quadrants are based on the intersection of the midline and the transverse line. Note that left and right are always in reference to the patient's left and right.

1. Left upper quadrant (LUQ)

2. Right upper quadrant (RUQ)

3. Left lower quadrant (LLQ)

4. Right lower quadrant (RLQ)

IV. **SKELETAL SYSTEM**

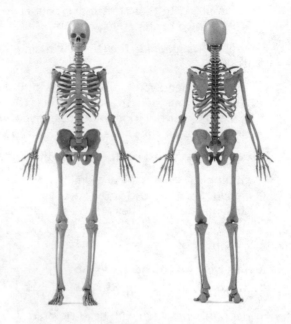

Figure 7.2

A. The skeletal system provides shape, allows movement, and protects internal organs.

B. There are 206 bones in the human body.

C. Tendons, ligaments, and cartilage are also part of the skeletal system.

    1. Ligaments connect bone to bone.

    2. Tendons connect bone muscle.

    3. Cartilage is connective tissue that allows smooth movement of joints.

D. Axial Skeleton. The axial skeleton consists primarily of the skull, spinal column, and rib cage (thoracic cavity).

    1. Skull

        i. Frontal bone: the forehead

  ii. Parietal bone: top of head, between frontal and occipital bones

  iii. Occipital bone: posterior portion of the skull

  iv. Temporal bone: lateral bones, above the cheekbones

  v. Maxillae: forms the upper jaw, above upper teeth

  vi. Mandible: movable portion of lower jaw

  vii. Zygomatic bone: cheekbones

  viii. Nasal bone: the nose

  ix. Foramen magnum: opening in the occipital bone where brain connects to spinal cord

2. Spinal column

  i. Central supporting structure; protects the spinal cord

  ii. Consists of 33 vertebrae (9 of them are fused)

  iii. The spinal column in descending order (superior to inferior):

   ➤ Cervical spine: 7 vertebrae, C1 to C7

   ➤ Thoracic spine: 12 vertebrae, T1 to T12

   ➤ Lumbar spine: 5 vertebrae, L1 to L5

   ➤ Sacrum: 5 fused vertebrae

   ➤ Coccyx: 4 fused vertebrae

3. Thoracic cavity

  i. Houses the heart, lungs, trachea, esophagus, and great vessels

  ii. Sternum: breastbone

   ➤ Manubrium: upper portion of the sternum

   ➤ Body: middle portion of the sternum

   ➤ Xiphoid process: inferior tip of the sternum

E. Appendicular Skeleton

1. Includes the bones of the arms, legs, and pelvis

2. Shoulder girdle: formed by the clavicle (collarbone), scapula (shoulder blade), humerus (upper arm)

3. Arm

    i.   Humerus: upper arm

    ii.   Radius: lateral bone of forearm (thumb side)

    iii. Ulna: medial bone of forearm

    iv. Carpal bones (wrist)

    v.   Metacarpals (base of the fingers)

    vi. Phalanges (fingers)

4. Pelvis: a ring-shaped structure formed by three bones

    i.   Illium: upper portion of the pelvis

    ii.   Ischium: lower portion of the pelvis

    iii. Pubis: anterior portion of the pelvis

5. Leg

    i.   Femur: thigh bone (the strongest bone of the body)

    ii.   Patella: kneecap

    iii. Tibia: medial bone of the lower leg (shinbone)

    iv. Fibula: lateral bone of the lower leg

    v.   Tarsal bones (ankle)

    vi. Metatarsal (base of the toes)

    vii. Phalanges (toes)

6. Joints. A joint exists where two long bones come together.

    i.   Symphysis: a joint with limited motion

    ii.   Ball-and-socket joint: a joint where the distal end is capable of free motion, such as the shoulder

    iii. Hinge joint: a joint where the bones can move only uniaxially, such as the knee

F. Muscles. There are three types of muscles.

1. Smooth muscle: involuntary muscle located within the blood vessels and the digestive tract

2. Skeletal: voluntary muscle that attaches to the skeleton

    i.   Biceps: anterior humerus

ii. Triceps: posterior humerus

iii. Pectoralis: anterior chest

iv. Latissimus dorsi: posterior chest

v. Rectus abdominis: abdominal muscles

vi. Quadriceps (four muscles): anterior femur

vii. Biceps femoris: posterior femur; part of hamstring muscle

viii. Gluteus (three muscles): buttocks

3. Cardiac: heart muscle

V. RESPIRATORY SYSTEM

A. The respiratory system provides the body with adequate oxygen and eliminates waste products such as carbon dioxide (CO_2). The respiratory system helps regulate pH levels to assist in maintaining homeostasis.

B. Upper Airway

1. Components of the upper airway include

   i. nose and mouth

   ii. nasopharynx (upper part of the throat behind the nose)

   iii. oropharynx (area of the throat behind the mouth)

   iv. larynx (voice box)

   v. epiglottis (valve that protects the opening of the trachea)

2. Most of the manual airway techniques and mechanical airway adjuncts used by the EMT are designed to clear and protect the upper airway.

3. Foreign-body airway obstruction (FBAO) is a concern for the EMT. The tongue is by far the most common cause of upper-airway obstruction.

C. Lower Airway

1. Components of lower airway include

   i. trachea

    ii. carina (where the trachea branches into left and right mainstem bronchi)

   iii. left and right mainstem bronchi (primary branches of the trachea leading to left and right lungs)

   iv. bronchioles (smaller branches of the bronchi)

    v. alveoli

➤ All airway structures above the alveoli serve to get air to this point in the respiratory system.

➤ This is the only place in the respiratory system where oxygen and carbon dioxide are exchanged.

➤ Alveoli are in contact with pulmonary capillaries.

➤ Pulmonary capillaries diffuse carbon dioxide from the body to the alveoli.

➤ Alveoli diffuse oxygen from the respiratory system to the body.

➤ Surfactant is a substance that helps keep the alveoli from collapsing.

D. Lung Expansion

  1. Pleura: two thin, smooth layers of tissue with thin film of fluid in between to allow frictionless movement across one another

    i. Visceral pleura: lines the outer surface of the lungs

   ii. Parietal pleura: lines the inside surface of the chest cavity

  2. During inhalation, as the chest expands, the parietal pleura pull the visceral pleura, which pull the lungs.

E. Muscles of Breathing

  1. Diaphragm

    i. The diaphragm is the primary muscle of respiration.

   ii. It separates the thoracic cavity from the abdominal cavity.

   iii. It is usually under involuntary control but can be controlled voluntarily.

   iv. The esophagus and great vessels pass through the diaphragm.

    v.   The diaphragm is dome shaped until it contracts during inhalation. During inhalation, it moves down and expands the size of the thoracic cavity.

2. Intercostal muscles. Located between the ribs, the intercostal muscles contract during inhalation and expand the thoracic cage.

3. Respiration and ventilation.

    i.   In general, the terms "respiration," "ventilation," and "breathing" refer to the movement of air in and out of the lungs. Although they are often used synonymously, there are some distinctions to be made. Ventilation is also called pulmonary ventilation.

    ii.   Inhalation through negative pressure breathing

       ➤ The diaphragm and intercostal muscles contract, the thoracic cage expands, pressure in the chest cavity decreases, and air rushes in.

       ➤ Inhalation is an active process and requires energy.

       ➤ Atmospheric air contains 21% oxygen.

    iii. Exhalation

       ➤ The diaphragm and intercostal muscles relax, the thoracic cage contracts, pressure in the chest cavity rises, and air is expelled.

       ➤ Exhalation is normally passive and does not require energy.

       ➤ Exhaled air contains 16% oxygen.

    iv. External respiration: the exchange of oxygen and carbon dioxide between the alveoli and pulmonary capillaries

    v.   Internal respiration: gas exchanged between the body's cells and the systemic capillaries

    vi. Cellular respiration (better known as aerobic metabolism): uses oxygen to break down glucose to create energy

F. Carbon Dioxide Drive

1. This is the primary mechanism of breathing control for most people.

2. The brain stem monitors carbon dioxide (CO_2) levels in the blood and cerebrospinal fluid.

3. High CO_2 levels will stimulate an increase in respiratory rate and tidal volume.

G. Hypoxic Drive

   1. Hypoxic drive is a backup system to the CO_2 drive.

   2. Specialized sensors in the brain, aorta, and carotid arteries monitor oxygen levels.

   3. Low oxygen levels will stimulate breathing.

   4. The hypoxic drive is less effective than CO_2 drive.

H. Lung Volumes

   1. Tidal volume: the amount of air inhaled or exhaled in one breath.

   2. Residual volume: amount of air in the lungs after completely exhaling. The residual volume keeps the lungs open.

   3. Inspiratory and expiratory reserve volume: the amount of air you can still inhale or exhale after a normal breath.

   4. Dead space: the amount of air in the respiratory system not including the alveoli.

   5. Minute volume: respiratory rate *x* tidal volume.

I. Normal Breathing

   1. Normal rate and tidal volume

      i. Normal adult rate: 12 to 20 breaths per minute (bpm)

      ii. Normal pediatric rate: 15 to 30 bpm

      iii. Normal infant rate: 25 to 50 bpm

   2. Non-labored

   3. Regular rhythm

   4. Clear and equal breath sounds bilaterally

J. Abnormal Breathing

   1. Abnormal rate or tidal volume

   2. Labored breathing

3. Muscle retractions

    i.   Intercostal retractions: between the ribs

    ii. Supraclavicular retractions: above the clavicles

    iii. Use of abdominal muscles

4. Abnormal skin color

5. Tripod position: seated, leaning forward, and using the arms to help breath

6. Agonal breaths: dying gasps; slow and shallow; will not move air into alveoli

VI. CIRCULATORY SYSTEM

A. The circulatory system includes all blood vessels, capillaries, and the heart. It is also called the cardiovascular system.

B. The Heart

1. A muscular organ with two pumps, one on the left side and another on the right

    i.   The left pump receives oxygenated blood from the lungs and sends it throughout the body. It is the stronger of the two pumps, with a greater workload than the right pump.

    ii. The right pump receives deoxygenated blood from the body and sends it to the lungs to drop off carbon dioxide and pick up oxygen on its way to the left heart.

    iii. A septal wall divides the heart into left and right sides.

2. Three layers of heart muscle and pericardium

    i.   Endocardium: smooth, thin lining on the inside of the heart

    ii. Myocardium: thick muscular wall of the heart

    iii. Epicardium: outermost layer of the heart and innermost layer of the pericardium

    iv. Pericardium: fibrous sac surrounding the heart

3. The chambers and valves

    i.   Atria: the two upper chambers of the heart. Blood returning to the heart on both sides enters the atria (atrium). The atria pump the blood into the ventricles just before the ventricles contract. This is called the "atrial kick" and helps increase cardiac output.

ii. Ventricles: the lower and larger chambers of the heart. Ventricles receive blood from the atria and send it out of the heart during ventricular contraction. Under normal circumstances, this generates a palpable pulse. The left ventricle sends oxygen-rich blood throughout the body under high pressure. The right ventricle sends oxygen-depleted blood to the lungs under low pressure.

iii. Heart valves: one-way valves between the atria and ventricles that allow blood to move in a downward direction into the ventricles during atrial contraction. The valves then close during ventricular contraction to prevent regurgitation of blood back into the atria.

4. Cardiac conduction system

i. The heart has its own electrical system. It generates electrical impulses, which stimulate contraction of the heart muscle.

ii. The heart can generate electrical impulses from three different locations. The primary power plant, the sinoatrial (SA) node, normally generates impulses between 60 to 100 times per minute in the adult. That's why the normal heart rate in adults is 60 to 100 beats per minute.

➤ The atrioventricular (AV) junction is the backup pacemaker and generates electrical impulses at about 40 to 60 per minute.

➤ The bundle of His is the final pacemaker for the heart. It generates impulses only at about 20 to 40 per minute.

iii. The heart, like the brain, is extremely intolerant of a lack of oxygen. The heart receives its blood flow from the coronary arteries, which branch off of the aorta.

iv. Cardiac output (circulation) will cease if the heart is unable to generate electrical impulses or if the heart muscle is too damaged to respond to the impulses.

5. Cardiac contraction

i. Myocardial contractility

➤ Contractility refers to the heart's ability to contract.

➤ Adequate contractility requires adequate blood volume and muscle strength.

ii. Preload

➤ Preload is the precontraction pressure based on the amount of blood coming back to the heart.

➤ Increased preload leads to increased stretching of the ventricles and increased myocardial contractility.

iii. Afterload

➤ Afterload is the resistance the heart must overcome during ventricular contraction.

➤ Increased afterload leads to decreased cardiac output.

The Pathway of Blood Flow Through the Heart

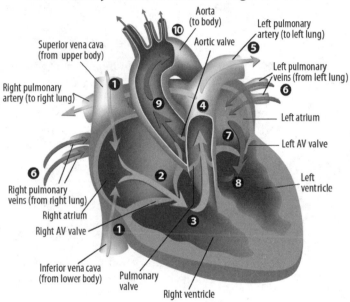

Figure 7.3

C. Blood Flow Through the Cardiovascular System

1. Oxygen-rich blood exits the left heart through the aorta. The aorta branches off into arteries, then arterioles, and finally capillaries. On the venous side, capillaries feed into venules, then veins, and finally the superior or inferior vena cava.

2. In Figure 7.3, the vena cava (1) returns blood to the right side of the heart into the right atrium (2). The right atrium pumps blood into the right ventricle (3), which pumps deoxygenated blood through the pulmonary arteries (4 and 5) into the lungs. The carbon dioxide and oxygen exchange takes place between the alveoli and the pulmonary capillaries. Oxygen-rich blood from the lungs returns to the left heart through the pulmonary veins (6) into the left atrium (7). The left atrium pumps blood into the left ventricle (8), which then pumps it to the aorta (9 and 10) for circulation throughout the body.

3. Arteries always carry blood away from the heart, and veins always carry blood toward the heart. Note the pulmonary artery is the one artery in the body that carries deoxygenated blood. The pulmonary vein is the only vein in the body that carries oxygen-rich blood.

4. Systemic vascular resistance (SVR)

   i. SVR is the resistance to blood flow throughout the body (excluding the pulmonary system).

   ii. SVR is determined by the size of blood vessels:

   ➤ Constriction (reduced size) of blood vessels increases SVR and can cause an increase in blood pressure.

   ➤ Dilation (increased size) of blood vessels decreases SVR and can lower blood pressure.

D. Arterial Pulses

   1. Central pulses

      i. Carotid pulse: can be felt by palpating the carotid artery in the neck during contraction of the left ventricle

      ii. Femoral: can be felt by palpating the femoral artery in the groin area during contraction of the left ventricle

   2. Peripheral pulses

      i. Radial pulse: palpated in the wrist on the radial (thumb) side

      ii. Brachial pulse: palpated on the medial portion of the upper arm beneath the biceps muscle; can also be felt on the anterior medial area of the arm where the humerus meets the forearm (elbow area)

      iii. Dorsalis pedis: palpated on top of the foot

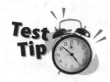

It takes a lot to memorize how blood flows through the circulatory system, including the heart's chambers and valves, but it is worth the effort! With this knowledge, you are likely to answer a few more questions correctly on the NREMT exam. You will also be better able to distinguish the signs of left heart failure from right heart failure in the field.

VII. BLOOD, BLOOD PRESSURE, AND PERFUSION

A. Components of Blood

1. Plasma: the liquid component of blood; made mostly of water

2. Red blood cells (erythrocytes): the oxygen-carrying component of blood

3. White blood cells (leukocytes): fight infection by defending against invading organisms

4. Platelets: essential for clot formation to stop bleeding

B. Blood Pressure. Blood pressure is a measurement of the pressure exerted against the walls of the arteries.

1. Systolic pressure: the blood pressure exerted during contraction of the left ventricle

2. Diastolic pressure: the blood pressure in between contractions

C. Perfusion. Perfusion is the flow of blood throughout the body.

1. Adequate perfusion means blood flow is adequate to all the tissues and organs in the body.

2. Inadequate perfusion (hypoperfusion or shock) means blood flow has been compromised to the point the entire body is at risk.

VIII. NERVOUS SYSTEM

A. Structural and Functional Divisions of the Nervous System

1. Central nervous system (CNS)

    i.   The CNS consists of the brain and spinal cord.

    ii. The CNS is the command and control portion of the nervous system.

   iii. The brain receives information from the peripheral nervous system (PNS), makes decisions, and sends orders to the PNS.

   iv. Parts of the brain

     ➤ Cerebrum: largest part of the brain; controls thought, memory, and the senses

     ➤ Cerebellum: coordinates voluntary movement, fine motor function, and balance

     ➤ Brain stem: includes midbrain, pons, and medulla; controls essential body functions, such as breathing and consciousness

   v. The spinal cord is the communication bridge between the brain and the PNS.

     ➤ Cerebrospinal fluid (CSF): a clear fluid in and around brain and spinal cord; cushions the CNS and filters contaminants

2. Peripheral nervous system

   i. The PNS includes all other nervous system structures outside of the CNS, including cranial and peripheral nerves.

   ii. The PNS sends information to the CNS and carries out orders from the CNS.

   iii. Two divisions of the PNS

     ➤ Sensory division: sends sensory information to the CNS.

     ➤ Motor division: receives motor commands from the CNS. There are two divisions of the motor portion of PNS.

       — Somatic: voluntary portion of the PNS

       — Autonomic nervous system (ANS): involuntary portion of the PNS

         a. Sympathetic: "fight or flight" portion of autonomic nervous system; exerts greater control in times of stress or danger

         b. Parasympathetic: "feed and breed" portion of nervous system; exerts greater control in times of rest, digestion, or reproduction

IX. INTEGUMENTARY SYSTEM (SKIN)

A. Epidermis

1. Outermost layer of the skin

2. Two epidermal layers

   i.   The germinal layer produces new cells and pushes them to the surface. The cells die en route to the surface.

   ii. The stratum corneal layer is the top epidermal layer and consists of dead skin cells.

3. Dermis. The dermis contains blood vessels, nerve endings, sweat glands, and hair follicles.

B. Subcutaneous Tissue

1. Fatty tissue

2. The deepest layer of the integumentary system, above the muscle layer

X. ABDOMINAL CAVITY

A. The abdominal cavity contains numerous organs of digestion and excretion.

B. It is separated from the thoracic cavity by the diaphragm.

C. It continues inferiorly into the pelvic cavity. The two continuous cavities are sometimes referred to as the abdominopelvic cavity.

D. The abdominal cavity is divided into four quadrants by the transverse line and the midline.

E. Organs

1. Esophagus: collapsible digestive structure running from mouth to stomach. The esophagus resides posterior to the trachea.

2. Stomach: hollow digestive organ in LUQ. The stomach receives food, begins breaking it down, and sends it to the small intestine.

3. Pancreas: solid organ. It aids in digestion, produces insulin, and helps regulate blood glucose levels.

4. Liver: solid organ; occupies most of the RUQ. The liver helps break down fats, filters toxins, and produces cholesterol.

5. Gall bladder: a hollow organ positioned beneath the liver. The gall bladder collects and stores bile from the liver. It releases bile into the intestine to aid in digestion.

6. Small intestine: hollow organ; occupies both lower abdominal quadrants. Food from the stomach is mixed with digestive enzymes to digest fat. Most of the contents are absorbed out of the small intestine and used or stored by the body.

7. Large intestine: hollow organ; includes the colon and rectum. Occupies the outer border of the abdomen. The large intestine pulls most of the remaining liquid to form solid stool.

8. Appendix: a hollow organ in the RLQ. It can become easily obstructed, causing inflammation, rupture, and life-threatening infection.

9. Spleen: a solid organ with little protection in the LUQ. The spleen filters the blood. It has a rich blood supply and can be a source of severe internal bleeding.

10. Kidneys: solid organs, part of the urinary system. The kidneys control fluid balance, filter waste, and control pH balance.

XI. ENDOCRINE SYSTEM

A. A system of glands that secrete hormones into the blood to help regulate body functions

B. Responsible for insulin production and regulation of blood glucose levels

XII. URINARY SYSTEM

A. Filters waste from the blood through the kidneys

B. Controls fluid balance in the body

C. Controls pH (acid-base balance) to maintain homeostasis

D. Ureters are tubes connecting each kidney to the bladder. Urine moves from the kidneys through the ureters into the bladder and then through the urethra and out of the body.

XIII. REPRODUCTIVE SYSTEM

A. Males: includes testicles, penis, and sperm. The prostate gland is part of the male reproductive system. It surrounds the urethra near the bladder.

B. Females: includes ovaries, fallopian tubes, and vagina.

XIV. CELLULAR ENERGY AND METABOLISM

A. Adenosine Triphosphate (ATP)

1. The body uses oxygen to convert nutrients into cellular energy called ATP.

2. Cells receive exponentially more ATP if there is an adequate oxygen supply.

B. Aerobic Metabolism

1. Aerobic metabolism is the creation of cellular energy with the use of oxygen. It is by far the most efficient means of energy production.

2. The heart and brain will cease function without an adequate supply of oxygen. The lungs and kidneys are also very sensitive to a lack of oxygen.

3. The waste products of aerobic metabolism are water and carbon dioxide. The human body is well equipped to handle these by-products through the respiratory and urinary systems.

C. Anaerobic Metabolism

1. Anaerobic metabolism is the creation of energy without an adequate oxygen supply. Much of the body (not the heart or brain) can switch over to an anaerobic metabolism when necessary.

2. The body will triage the oxygen supply when necessary, sending it to the most critical areas and forcing other areas into an anaerobic state.

3. The by-products of anaerobic metabolism include lactic acid. The body needs much longer to deal with by-products of anaerobic metabolism and cannot complete the process until adequate oxygen supply is restored.

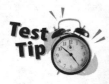

Compared to the previous EMT training curriculum, the current National EMS Education Standards place a stronger emphasis on anatomy, physiology, pathophysiology, and terminology. This emphasis will definitely be reflected on the national certification exam. Be sure to study the material in this chapter.

XV. INFANTS AND CHILDREN

A. Anatomical Differences from Adults

1. The pediatric tongue is larger in proportion to the airway.

2. The pediatric airway is more easily obstructed.

3. The pediatric head is larger in proportion to the body.

Author's Note: *The internet is replete with illustrations of the anatomical structures and systems presented in this chapter. If you are struggling with any of the information presented in this chapter, I recommend you do an internet search for "images of . . . ."*

PRACTICE QUESTIONS

1. Which of the following regarding homeostasis is correct?

   A. Homeostasis is a state of balance or equilibrium within the body.

   B. Homeostasis is assured if all vital signs are within normal limits.

   C. The body works to avoid homeostasis over prolonged periods.

   D. Patients who are alert and without pain are demonstrating homeostasis.

2. The frontal plane divides the body into

   A. left and right sides.

   B. top and bottom halves.

   C. anterior and posterior.

   D. proximal and distal.

3. From anatomical position, which of the following is the lateral bone in the forearm?

   A. the ulna

   B. the radius

   C. the humerus

   D. the tibia

4. Ventral refers to the

   A. anterior surface.

   B. posterior surface.

   C. medial aspect.

   D. lateral aspect.

5. Your adult patient is unconscious, breathing adequately, and has a pulse. There is no indication of trauma. The patient should be positioned

   A. in the shock position.

   B. supine.

   C. prone.

   D. recovery position.

ANSWERS

1. A.

   Homeostasis is a state of balance or equilibrium within the body. The body works to constantly maintain homeostasis.

2. C.

The frontal plane divides the body into anterior and posterior. The transverse plane divides the body into superior and inferior. The midline divides the body into left and right.

3. B.

The radius is the lateral bone in the forearm. The ulna is the medial bone in the forearm. The humerus is in the upper arm. The tibia is the medial bone in the lower leg.

4. A.

Ventral refers to the anterior surface. Dorsal refers to the posterior surface.

5. D.

The patient should be placed in the recovery position to help protect the airway. The shock position (Trendelenburg) is no longer recommended.

Life Span Development

I. INFANTS

A. Ages

    1. Neonate: a newborn from birth to one month of age

    2. Infant: up to one year of age

B. Vital Signs

    1. Respirations. Normal respiratory rate is about 30 to 60 breaths per minute (bpm) for newborns and about 25 to 50 bpm for infants.

    2. Pulse. Normal pulse rate is about 140 to 160 beats per minute for newborns and about 100 to 140 beats per minute for infants.

    3. Blood pressure. A newborn's blood pressure is about 70 systolic and will increase to about 90 systolic by one year of age.

C. Physiology

    1. The typical newborn weight is about 6 to 8 pounds (3 to 3.5 kilograms). The newborn's weight will typically double by six months and triple by about one year.

    2. The newborn's head makes up about 25% of the body and is a significant source of heat loss.

    3. During the first couple weeks, neonates often lose weight, and then begin to gain it back.

    4. The newborn's fontanelles (soft spots on the skull) will be fully fused by about 18 months. Depressed fontanelles may indicate hypovolemia.

    5. Infants are often nose breathers and can develop respiratory distress easily.

6. Rapid breathing can lead to fluid loss and loss of body heat.

7. Hyperventilation of infants presents significant risk of barotrauma.

D. Neonates typically have

1. startle reflex: opens arms wide, spreading fingers

2. grip reflex: grips when something placed in palm

3. rooting reflex: turns toward a touch to the cheek

4. sucking reflex: stimulated by touching the lips

E. Infants

1. At 6 months: typically begin teething, can sit upright, and track objects visually

2. At 12 months

   i. Typically know their name, recognize parents or caregivers, walk with assistance, and speak a few words

   ii. Still communicate distress primarily through crying

II. TODDLERS AND PRESCHOOLERS

A. Age

1. Toddlers: one to three years old

2. Preschoolers: three to six years old

B. Vitals

1. Toddlers

   i. Respirations: about 20 to 30 bpm

   ii. Heart rate: about 90 to 140 beats per minute

   iii. Blood pressure: about 80 to 90 systolic

2. Preschoolers

   i. Respirations: about 20 to 25 bpm

   ii. Heart rate: 80 to 130 beats per minute

   iii. Blood pressure: about 90 to 110 systolic

C. Physiology

    1. As the immune system develops, children at this age typically experience a number of minor colds, viruses, flu-like symptoms, respiratory infections, etc.

    2. Fine motor skills improve, and the brain grows rapidly in size.

D. Toddlers typically walk, climb, distinguish basic shapes and colors, and are potty trained.

E. Preschoolers typically

    1. are physically coordinated and communicate well verbally

    2. know their name and address and can dress themselves

    3. can count to 10 or beyond

F. Recommendations

    1. Separation anxiety is common. Allow child to stay with caregiver when possible.

    2. Communicate directly with the child, not just the caregivers.

    3. Choose your words carefully. They will probably be taken literally.

    4. Do not lie.

III. SCHOOL-AGE CHILDREN: 6 TO 12 YEARS OLD

A. Vitals

    1. Respirations: about 15 to 20 bpm

    2. Heart rate: 70 to 110 beats per minute

    3. Blood pressure: about 90 to 120 systolic

B. Physiology

    1. Permanent teeth replace baby teeth.

    2. The musculoskeletal system is growing rapidly.

C. School-age children typically

    1. read and write

2. develop basic problem-solving skills

3. are establishing their self-image and morals

4. have a large social circle due to school

5. understand the concept of death

6. look up to authority figures such as police officers and firefighters

D. Recommendations

1. Communicate in understandable terms, but do not talk down to them.

2. Respect the privacy rights for this age group.

 ## IV. ADOLESCENTS: 12 TO 18 YEARS OF AGE

A. Vitals

1. Respirations: 12 to 20 bpm

2. Heart rate: 60 to 100 beats per minute

3. Blood pressure: about 100 to 120 systolic

B. Physiology

1. Significant physical growth occurs over about a three-year period.

2. Eating disorders are more common in this age group.

3. Puberty occurs.

C. Adolescents often

1. exhibit argumentative behavior, and are hypercritical and egocentric

2. do not anticipate the consequences of their actions

3. are subject to a great deal of peer pressure, and are at higher risk for depression and suicide

4. are preoccupied with body image and physical appearance

5. become sexually active

D. Recommendation: For sensitive matters, talk with the adolescent without caregivers present when possible.

V. ADULTHOOD

A. Stages of Adulthood

   1. Early adulthood: 20 to 40 years of age

   2. Middle adulthood: 40 to 60 years of age

   3. Late adulthood: over 60 years of age

B. Vitals

   1. Respirations: 12 to 20 bpm

   2. Heart rate: 60 to 100 beats per minute

   3. Blood pressure: about 110/70 to 130/90

C. Characteristics

   1. Accidental trauma is a leading cause of death in the young adult age group.

   2. Mild physical decline typically develops in the middle adult age group.

   3. Women typically experience menopause during middle adulthood.

   4. Continued physical and mental decline is common in late adulthood.

   5. Older adults frequently have extensive medical histories and are on multiple medications.

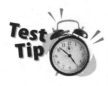

Test Tip

Priority-of-treatment *questions are common on the certification exam. These questions often end with "Your next action should be . . . "or "Your first action should be . . . " Expect questions that challenge you to select the most important action or the next correct action for a given scenario. Knowing the NREMT trauma and medical assessment skill sheets will be extremely helpful. If you know the order of assessments and interventions on the skill sheets, you are more likely to identify the correct answers on the test.*

PRACTICE QUESTIONS

1. While assessing an infant, you note depressed fontanelles. This indicates that the infant

   A. is most likely dehydrated.

   B. is perfusing normally.

   C. has increased intracranial pressure.

   D. has been crying recently.

2. Your patient is two years old. She would be considered a(n)

   A. neonate.

   B. infant.

   C. toddler.

   D. preschooler.

3. To ease a child's anxiety, it is usually best to

   A. transport rapidly.

   B. isolate the child.

   C. avoid eye contact.

   D. keep caregivers close by.

4. Eating disorders are more common among which of the following age groups?

   A. adolescents

   B. school age

   C. toddlers

   D. older adults

5. Which of the following statements is correct?

   A. Mild physical decline typically develops in the young adult age group.

   B. Women typically experience menopause during early adulthood.

   C. Physical and mental acuity peaks in late adulthood.

   D. Accidental trauma is a leading cause of death in the young adult age group.

ANSWERS

1. **A.**

   Depressed fontanelles indicate probable hypovolemia, usually due to dehydration. Bulging fontanelles would indicate increased intracranial pressure.

2. **C.**

   From birth to one month is a neonate. An infant is up to one year. Toddlers are from one to three years and preschoolers are from three to six years.

3. **D.**

   Separation anxiety is common. Allow children to stay with caregivers when possible.

4. **A.**

   Eating disorders are more common in the adolescent age group.

5. **D.**

   Accidental trauma is a leading cause of death in the young adult age group.

PART III

AIRWAY, PHARMACOLOGY, AND PATIENT ASSESSMENT

Airway, Respiration, and Artificial Ventilation

Note: Before proceeding with this chapter, be sure to see Chapter 7 for a review of the upper and lower airways.

I. PHYSIOLOGY OF BREATHING

A. Ventilation

1. Ventilation is the moving of air in and out of the lungs.

2. Ventilation is required for effective oxygenation and respiration.

3. Inhalation is the active part of ventilation. Energy is required.

   i. During inhalation, the diaphragm and intercostal muscles contract, intrathoracic pressure decreases, and a vacuum is created.

   ii. As the thorax enlarges, air passes through the upper airway into the lower airway and finally into the alveoli.

4. Exhalation

   i. Exhalation is the passive part of ventilation. No energy is required.

   ii. During exhalation, the diaphragm and intercostal muscles relax, the thorax decreases in size, and air is compressed out of the lungs.

   iii. During exhalation, intrathoracic pressure exceeds atmospheric pressure.

5. Airway obstruction

   i. Airway obstruction (blockage of an airway structure leading to the alveoli) will prevent effective ventilation.

   ii. Causes of airway obstruction include

     ➤ tongue (the number one cause of airway obstruction)

     ➤ fluid (saliva, blood, mucus, vomit, etc.)

     ➤ swelling

     ➤ foreign bodies (food, toys, etc.)

6. Regulation of ventilation

   i. The need for oxygen can rise or fall based on activity, illness, injury, etc. The primary methods of controlling oxygen delivery are

     ➤ increasing or decreasing the rate of breathing

     ➤ increasing or decreasing the tidal volume of breaths

   ii. Hypoxia

     ➤ Inadequate delivery of oxygen to the cells

     ➤ Early indications of hypoxia: restlessness, anxiety, irritability, dyspnea, tachycardia

     ➤ Late indications of hypoxia: altered or decreased level of consciousness, severe dyspnea, cyanosis, and bradycardia (especially in pediatric patients)

   iii. The carbon dioxide drive

     ➤ The carbon dioxide (CO_2) drive is the body's primary system for monitoring breathing status.

     ➤ The body monitors CO_2 levels in the blood and cerebrospinal fluid.

   iv. Hypoxic drive

     ➤ The hypoxic drive is a backup system to the CO_2 drive.

     ➤ It monitors oxygen levels in plasma.

     ➤ It may be used by end-stage chronic obstructive pulmonary disease (COPD) patients who have chronically high levels of CO_2.

➤ Prolonged exposure to high concentrations of oxygen in hypoxic-drive patients may depress spontaneous ventilations.

➤ Withholding oxygen from acutely ill or injured patients is *not* recommended.

B. Oxygenation

1. Oxygenation is delivery of oxygen to the blood.

2. Ventilation is required for oxygenation.

3. Oxygenation is required for respiration but does not ensure respiration.

4. Ventilation does not ensure oxygenation. For example, in cases of smoke inhalation and carbon monoxide poisoning, ventilation occurred, but not oxygenation.

5. Surrounding air contains about 21% oxygen. Expired air contains about 16% oxygen.

C. Respiration

1. Respiration is the exchange of oxygen and carbon dioxide.

2. Time and injury

i. The heart and brain become irritable due to lack of oxygen almost immediately.

ii. Brain damage begins within about 4 minutes.

iii. Permanent brain damage likely within 6 minutes.

iv. Irrecoverable injury is likely within 10 minutes.

II. ASSESSMENT

A. Assessment of breathing includes looking, listening, and feeling.

1. Look for chest rise and fall.

2. Listen for breathing, ability to speak, lung sounds.

3. Feel for air movement and chest rise and fall. Place your ear near the victim's mouth and nose, and your hand on the victim's chest.

B. Adequate Breathing

1. Normal respiratory rate and rhythm

    i.   Adults: about 12 to 20 breaths per minute (bpm)

    ii. Children: about 15 to 30 bpm

    iii. Infants: about 25 to 50 bpm

2. Nonlabored breathing

3. Adequate tidal volume (chest rise and fall)

4. Clear bilateral lung sounds

C. Inadequate Breathing

1. Abnormal respiratory rate or breathing pattern

2. Nasal flaring (enlargement of the nostrils during breathing)

3. Abnormal, diminished, or absent lung sounds

4. Paradoxical motion (flail chest segment moves in opposite direction of the thorax)

5. Unequal rise and fall of the chest

6. Dyspnea, accessory muscle use, retractions

7. Cyanosis

8. Agonal respiration (dying gasps), or apnea (no breathing).

D. Auscultation of Lung Sounds

1. Auscultation is the use of a stethoscope to listen for lung sounds.

2. The top left lung field is compared to top right lung field. Same for mid- and lower lung fields. Lung sounds are compared side to side, not top to bottom.

3. Anterior auscultation

    i.   Place the stethoscope at the midclavicular line about the second intercostal space. This is about 2 inches below the clavicle but above the nipple line. Auscultate bilaterally (on both sides of the chest).

    ii. Place the stethoscope at about the fourth intercostal space at the midaxillary line. This is below the armpit at about the nipple line. Auscultate bilaterally.

4. Posterior auscultation

    i. Lungs sounds are often easier to access or hear on the patient's posterior chest.

    ii. Place the stethoscope at about the midclavicular line above and below the scapula bilaterally.

5. Auscultate for lung sounds and equality.

    i. Normal lung sounds are clear and equal bilaterally.

    ii. Abnormal lung sounds

       ➤ Absent or diminished: indicates little or no air exchange.

       ➤ Wheezing: high-pitched sounds usually heard during exhalation.

       ➤ Rales: "wet" or "crackling" sounds.

       ➤ Stridor: a high-pitched sound indicating partial upper airway obstruction. Stridor is auscultated in the upper airway (neck), not the lower lung fields.

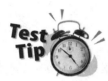

Test Tip

Remember that lung sounds are an important component when assessing a patient. Always auscultate lung sounds. This is especially important with respiratory patients, cardiac patients, significant trauma patients, any patient on supplemental oxygen, and any patient receiving artificial ventilations.

E. Pulse Oximetry

1. Considered the "sixth vital sign." Monitoring of oxygen saturation (SaO_2) is now part of the standard of care for EMS. Often a function provided on cardiac monitor/defibrillators.

2. SaO_2 measures the percentage of hemoglobin (red blood cells) that is saturated with oxygen. It does *not* identify definitively how much oxygen is in the blood; however, it is an indication of respiratory efficiency.

3. Normal SaO_2 is 98% or above. Below 94% indicates the need for supplemental oxygen.

4. Advantages of pulse oximetry: fast, easy, noninvasive assessment tool.

5. Limitations of pulse oximetry

   i. It is an indication of respiratory efficiency, not confirmation.

   ii. Pulse oximetry cannot measure the amount of hemoglobin, only the oxygen saturation of the hemoglobin that is present.

   iii. Other clinical assessments must be performed as well.

   iv. A measurement may be difficult to obtain on some patients due to hypovolemia, hypothermia, anemia, nail polish, carbon monoxide poisoning.

   v. Pulse oximetry measures saturation of hemoglobin; it cannot distinguish between oxygen saturation and carbon monoxide saturation.

   vi. There can be a time delay between the patient's pulse oximeter reading and the patient's current respiratory status.

III. INTERVENTIONS

A. Airway Management Skills

1. Manual airway techniques

   i. Manual airway techniques are used to open the airway, allow for suctioning, and prevent the tongue from obstructing the airway.

   ii. Head tilt–chin lift

     ➤ The preferred manual method of opening the airway

     ➤ Indication

       — Patients with altered or decreased level of consciousness

       — Patients with suspected airway obstruction

       — Patients requiring suctioning

     ➤ Contraindication (should not be used): suspected cervical-spine (c-spine) injury

   iii. Jaw-thrust maneuver

     ➤ Indication: patients with altered or decreased level of consciousness and suspected c-spine injury

     ➤ Contraindication: conscious patients

2. Mechanical airway adjuncts

    i.   Oropharyngeal airway (OPA)

- Used to prevent the tongue from obstructing the airway. Failure to size or insert OPA correctly can cause the tongue to block the airway.

- Indication: unresponsive patients without a gag reflex.

- Contraindications: conscious patients or any patient with an intact gag reflex.

- Sizing the OPA. Measure from the corner of the mouth to the earlobe. The OPA should be positioned during measurement as it will reside upon insertion.

- Inserting the OPA in Adults

 — Manually open the airway; suction as needed.

 — Insert OPA upside down with distal end pointing toward roof of mouth.

 — Rotate 180 degrees while advancing OPA until flange (flat proximal portion) rests on the patient's lips.

- Inserting the OPA in Pediatric Patients

 — Manually open the airway; suction as needed.

 — Depress tongue with a tongue depressor and insert directly (no rotation), or insert OPA sideways and rotate 90 degrees until flange rests on the lips.

- Remove the OPA immediately if the patient gags.

- Always have suction immediately available.

    ii.   Nasopharyngeal airway (NPA)

- Used to prevent the tongue from obstructing the airway in patients who may not be able to protect their own airway

- Indications

 — Unresponsive patients without a gag reflex

 — Patients with a decreased level of consciousness, but with an intact gag preventing use of the OPA

➤ Contraindications

— Conscious patients with an intact gag reflex capable of protecting their own airway

— Severe head injury or facial trauma

— Resistance to insertion in both nostrils

— NPAs are not typically used for patients under about one year of age.

➤ Sizing the NPA. Measure from the tip of the nose to the earlobe. The NPA should be positioned during measurement as it will reside upon insertion.

➤ Inserting the NPA

— Lubricate the NPA with a water-soluble lubricant prior to insertion. Do *not* use petroleum-based products.

— Always insert NPA with bevel toward the septum.

— Try larger nostril first. Switch if resistance is met.

— Advance gently, rotating as necessary, until flange rests against the nostril. Do *not* force NPA.

— Remove immediately if the patient begins to gag.

— Always have suction immediately available.

— If resistance is met upon insertion in both nostrils, discontinue use.

3. Suctioning

i. Aspiration (entry of matter into the lungs) drastically increases the risk of death.

ii. Suction is indicated if there are secretions (blood, vomit, mucus, oral secretions, etc.) in the airway that could be aspirated, obstruct the airway, or interfere with ventilations or insertion of a mechanical airway adjunct.

iii. Larger substances that cannot be suctioned (debris, foreign bodies, teeth, undigested food, etc.) should be removed manually.

iv. Suction should generally be performed after the airway is opened manually and before insertion of a mechanical airway adjunct.

v. Suction units

➤ All suction units should have a disposable suction canister.

➤ Portable and fixed suction units should be able to generate a vacuum of 300 mmHg when tubing is clamped.

➤ Portable suction: can be carried to the patient.

➤ Fixed suction: suction unit permanently mounted in vehicle, hospital, etc.

➤ Hand-powered suction: manually powered portable suction unit.

vi. Suction catheters

➤ A suction catheter attaches to the suction unit and is inserted into the patient's airway to remove secretions.

➤ Suction catheters, tubing, and disposable canisters are all single-patient use only.

➤ Rigid suction catheter

— Also known as a "tonsil tip" or Yankauer

— Best suited for suctioning the oral airway

➤ French catheter

— Also known as whistle-tip, a flexible catheter that comes in several sizes

— Best suited for suctioning the nose, stoma, or the inside of an advanced airway device

vii. Suction procedures

➤ Suctioning increases the risk of hypoxia. Suction time cannot exceed

— 15 seconds for adults

— 10 seconds for pediatric patients

— 5 seconds for infants

➤ Insert rigid suction catheter only as far as you can see.

➤ For French catheter, measure from corner of the mouth to the earlobe.

➤ Apply suction upon withdrawal of the catheter.

> ➤ Rinse the suction catheter and tubing with water after use to reduce risk of obstruction.

4. Recovery position

   i.   The recovery position (patient positioned on his side) reduces the risk of aspiration.

   ii. Unresponsive patients with adequate breathing and no c-spine injury should be placed in the recovery position.

B. Supplemental Oxygen

1. The goal of supplemental oxygen is to maintain a pulse oximetry reading of at least 94%.

   i.   Supplemental oxygen is not needed if there are no signs or symptoms of respiratory distress and the pulse oximetry is at least 94%.

   ii. When oxygen is administered, it should be titrated to maintain a pulse oximeter reading of at least 94%.

   iii. This approach to prehospital oxygen administration represents a fundamental shift in standards and philosophy.

2. Indications

   i.   Any patient in cardiac arrest

   ii.   Any patient receiving artificial ventilation

   iii. Any patient with suspected hypoxia

   iv.   Any patient with signs of shock (hypoperfusion)

   v.   Any patient with a pulse oximetry (SaO2) reading below 94%.

   vi.   Any patient with a medical condition or traumatic injury that may benefit from supplemental oxygen

   vii. Any patient with an altered or decreased level of consciousness

   viii. Contraindication: unsafe environment

3. Oxygen cylinders

   i.   Oxygen cylinders are seamless steel or aluminum cylinders of various sizes.

   > ➤ D cylinder: about 350-liter capacity

   > ➤ E cylinder: about 625-liter capacity

> ➤ M cylinder: about 3,000-liter capacity

> ➤ G cylinder: about 5,000-liter capacity

> ➤ H cylinder: about 7,000-liter capacity

ii. A green cylinder indicates that it contains oxygen.

iii. Cylinders should be safety tested every three to five years.

iv. Oxygen cylinders should never be left standing unattended.

v. The pin indexing system is a safety feature that prevents a carbon dioxide cylinder from being connected to an oxygen regulator.

vi. The amount of oxygen in a cylinder is measured in pounds per square inch (psi).

> ➤ A full cylinder is about 2,000 psi.

> ➤ The cylinder should be taken out of service and refilled if below 200 psi.

vii. Flow meters/pressure regulators. Flow meters are connected to pressure regulators. In combination, they reduce the pressure coming from the tank to safe levels and allow a specific flow rate. The flow rate is measured in liters per minute (lpm or L/min).

4. Nonrebreather (NRB) masks

i. Usually the preferred method of oxygen administration in prehospital

ii. Referred to as "high-flow" oxygen administration

iii. Available in adult and pediatric sizes

iv. Flow rate: 10 to 15 lpm

v. Oxygen delivered: up to 90%

vi. Cautions

> ➤ The reservoir must be full before applying mask to patient.

> ➤ Never administer less than 10 lpm.

> ➤ If the reservoir completely deflates during inhalation, the flow rate must be increased.

> ➤ Immediately remove mask if oxygen source is lost.

5. Nasal cannula

    i.   Referred to as "low-flow" oxygen administration

    ii.   Indications

        ➤ Patient will not tolerate a NRB.

        ➤ Patient is on long-term oxygen therapy via nasal cannula and there is no indication high-flow oxygen is needed.

    iii. Flow rate: 1 to 6 lpm

    iv.   Oxygen delivered: 24% to 44%. The nasal cannula delivers about 4% per liter.

    v.   Caution. Prolonged use can dry and irritate nasal passages if oxygen is not humidified.

6. Simple face mask

    i.   The simple face mask is similar to a nonrebreather, but without the oxygen reservoir.

    ii.   With a flow rate of 6 to 10 lpm, the simple face mask delivers 40% to 60% oxygen.

    iii. These are rarely used in the prehospital environment.

7. Venturi mask

    i.   A mask that delivers precise concentration of low-flow oxygen

    ii.   Rarely used in the prehospital environment

8. Supplemental oxygen in patients with a tracheostomy or stoma

    i.   A tracheostomy is a surgical procedure that creates an opening through the neck into the trachea.

    ii.   Stoma: a surgical opening into the trachea.

    iii. Patients with a tracheostomy ventilate through their stoma, not the mouth or nose. Supplemental oxygen should be applied over the stoma using a tracheostomy mask (not common in the prehospital environment) or a nonrebreather mask.

9. Humidification of oxygen

    i.   Humidification increases the moisture of supplemental oxygen by flowing it through water prior to inhalation by the patient.

    ii.   This technique is not often used in the prehospital setting.

10. Hazards of oxygen administration

   i. Combustible

      ➤ Oxygen supports combustion. High concentrations of oxygen accelerate combustion.

      ➤ Oxygen should be used only in a safe environment: no open flames, no cigarettes, etc.

   ii. Pressurized gas

      ➤ Oxygen cylinders contain a highly compressed gas and should be treated with great caution.

      ➤ Never leave an oxygen cylinder standing unattended. It should be routinely placed on its side and secured during transport.

   iii. Oxygen toxicity

      ➤ The alveoli can collapse due to long-term exposure to high concentrations of oxygen.

      ➤ Oxygen toxicity rarely occurs in prehospital environment.

   iv. Respiratory depression

      ➤ Respiratory depression is a risk for COPD patients on the hypoxic drive; however, it typically requires long-term exposure to high-concentration oxygen

      ➤ Retinal damage can occur in newborns with long-term exposure to high-concentration oxygen.

C. Assisted Ventilation

  1. Also called artificial ventilation or positive pressure ventilation (PPV), assisted ventilations includes

   i. mouth to mask

   ii. flow-restricted, oxygen-powered ventilation device and automatic transport ventilators (preference is region specific)

   iii. bag valve mask (BVM): two-person BVM, rather than one-person, is preferred

   iv. mouth to mouth

      ➤ Not a preferred method

      ➤ Continuous positive airway pressure (CPAP) device: used in special circumstances

2. Artificial ventilations are indicated for any patient with inadequate spontaneous breathing leading to severe respiratory distress or respiratory failure. This could be caused by

    i.   central nervous system injury, disease, or impairment

    ii. foreign-body airway obstruction

    iii. chest trauma, such as a flail chest or sucking chest wound

    iv. increased airway resistance due to bronchoconstriction, pulmonary edema, or inflammation

3. Patients requiring artificial ventilations are often unresponsive, but not always. Conscious patients can also need assistance due to severe respiratory distress or respiratory failure. In all cases, patients requiring artificial ventilations will demonstrate one of the following:

    i.   Apnea: no spontaneous breathing

    ii. Agonal breaths: shallow, ineffective gasps

    iii. Bradypnea: slow breathing

    iv. Tachypnea: fast breathing

    v.   Hypoventilation: breathing too slow or too shallow

4. Not every patient with bradypnea or tachypnea needs artificial ventilations. The indication for artificial ventilations is inadequate spontaneous breathing. Assess the patient for other signs of inadequate breathing, such as work of breathing, level of consciousness, skin color. When in doubt, begin artificial ventilations.

5. Consider providing artificial ventilations for any patient breathing less than 8 times per minute.

6. Consider providing artificial ventilations for any adult patient breathing more than 24 times per minute.

7. Any unresponsive patient receiving artificial ventilations should have an airway adjunct (OPA, NPA, etc.) in place to prevent the tongue from obstructing the airway.

8. Spontaneous breathing versus artificial ventilations

    i.   Normal spontaneous breathing is done through negative pressure.

    ii. Artificial ventilations are accomplished through positive pressure ventilations (PPV).

➤ Complications of PPV

— Increased intrathoracic pressure, which reduces circulatory efficiency

— Gastric distention, which increases the risk of vomiting and can compromise ventilatory efficiency

a. Use of the Sellick maneuver (also called cricoid pressure) is no longer recommended by the American Heart Association as a means to reduce gastric distention during artificial ventilation.

b. The Sellick maneuver should never be used during active vomiting.

➤ Hyperventilation

— Hyperventilation is a common mistake in the prehospital setting and must be avoided.

— Hyperventilation occurs when ventilations are provided too fast, too deep, or both.

— Risks of hyperventilation include circulatory and ventilatory compromise; gastric distention due to esophageal opening; vomiting and aspiration; and barotrauma, such as pneumothorax.

9. Appropriate rates and volumes of artificial ventilations

i. Correct tidal volume

➤ The best way to determine appropriate tidal volume is rise and fall of the chest.

— Artificial ventilations should cause gentle chest rise and fall.

— It should take at least 1 second to inflate the chest.

ii. Correct rates of artificial ventilation for apneic patients with a pulse

➤ Adults: one breath every 5 to 6 seconds (10 to 12 times per minute)

➤ Infants and children: one breath every 3 to 5 seconds (12 to 20 times per minute)

➤ Newborns: one breath every 1 to 1½ seconds (40 to 60 times per minute)

      iii.   In most cases, ventilations for patients in cardiac arrest are not based on the clock, they are based on the compression-to-ventilation ratio.

- ➤ 30 compressions: 2 breaths
  - — Always for adults
  - — Always for single-rescuer CPR on any patient
- ➤ 15 compressions: 2 breaths
  - — Two-rescuer CPR on children and infants
- ➤ 3 compressions: 1 breath
  - — Newborns
- ➤ It is not necessary to pause compressions for ventilations once an advanced airway has been placed. For patients in cardiac arrest with an advanced airway, provide one breath every 6 to 8 seconds (8 to 10 breaths per minute).

10.   Barrier device

    i.   A barrier device is a mask or shield placed between the victim's mouth and yours during artificial ventilations.

    ii.   Advantages

- ➤ The device is small and portable.
- ➤ It is easy to use effectively.
- ➤ It is safer than mouth-to-mouth when used with a one-way valve.
  - — One-way valve prevents secretions and exhaled air from traveling back up into the rescuer's mouth.
- ➤ Because barrier devices are easy to use, they are a preferred method of providing artificial ventilations. Expect to be asked a question about this on your certification exam!

    iii.   Disadvantage: delivers only about 16% oxygen (unless connected to supplemental oxygen)

11. Bag valve mask (BVM) device

    i.   The BVM is the most frequently used method of artificial ventilations in the prehospital setting.

ii. Advantages

> ➤ When used effectively with supplemental oxygen at about 15 lpm, the patient receives nearly 100% oxygen.

> ➤ Use of BVMs reduces biohazard risk for rescuers.

> ➤ Self-inflating BVMs do not need an oxygen source to function.

> ➤ Can be used with a mask or an advanced airway device.

iii. Disadvantages

> ➤ Single rescuers typically deliver less tidal volume with the BVM than with a barrier device.

> ➤ Effective use of a BVM by a single rescuer is highly difficult.

iv. Volumes for BVM devices

> ➤ Adult BVM: 1,200 to 1,600 mL

> ➤ Child BVM: 500 to 700 mL

> ➤ Infant BVM: 150 to 240 mL

v. Components of a BVM

> ➤ Self-inflating bag, single-patient use

> ➤ Clear mask, single-patient use, appropriately sized

> ➤ Oxygen reservoir

> ➤ One-way, non-jam inlet valve with standard fitting for face mask or advanced airway device

> ➤ Pop-off valves are *not* typically recommended for prehospital use.

vi. Single-rescuer BVM technique

> ➤ *Note*: Single-rescuer BVM is *not* a preferred technique.

> ➤ The rescuer must control the mask, mask seal, and head position with one hand and squeeze the bag with the other.

> ➤ The "EC" clamp technique is recommended for single-rescuer BVM usage.

>> — Thumb and index finger make a "C" around the mask.

— The remaining three fingers form an "E" and are placed along the angle of the jaw.

— The hand controlling the mask should be placed on the same side of the patient's jaw. In other words, the right hand of the rescuer controls the mask with the "E" on the patient's right jaw, or the left hand of rescuer controls mask with the "E" on the patient's left jaw.

— Search Internet for "images of EC clamp technique."

   vii. Two-rescuer BVM technique

➤ Two-person BVM is a preferred technique.

➤ One rescuer uses both hands to control the mask seal. This makes it considerably easier to maintain a good seal during ventilations.

➤ The other rescuer uses both hands to squeeze the bag. This makes it considerably easier to ventilate slowly, control tidal volume, and reduce gastric distention.

12. Manually triggered ventilation devices

   i. Also known as flow-restricted oxygen-powered ventilation devices (FROPVD).

   ii. Advantage: allows the rescuer to use a two-handed mask seal during artificial ventilations

   iii. Disadvantages

➤ Increased risk of gastric distention.

➤ Increased risk of barotrauma with infants and children.

➤ Numerous contraindications, such as COPD, chest trauma.

➤ Unable to feel bag mask compliance.

— Bag mask compliance is the "feel" of the bag during ventilations.

— Bag mask compliance is helpful in assessing ventilatory efficiency.

➤ Uses oxygen three to five times faster than manual bag valve mask ventilation.

➤ Device has a pressure-relief valve and may not effectively ventilate patients that require higher pressures.

13. Automatic transport ventilators (ATV)

    i. ATVs are similar to manually triggered ventilators, but the rate and tidal volume can be automated.

    ii. Advantages

        ➤ An ATV provides very consistent rates and tidal volumes, which can reduce risk of hyperventilation.

        ➤ An ATV allows the rescuer to use a two-handed mask seal, or frees hands entirely if advanced airway is in place.

    iii. Disadvantages

        ➤ Rescuer is unable to assess bag mask compliance.

        ➤ Additional training is required to safely calculate correct tidal volume.

            — Tidal volume based on 6 to 7 mL per kilogram of body weight

            — Tidal volume based on "ideal" body weight

        ➤ Incorrect rate or tidal volume can cause barotraumas or hypoventilation.

        ➤ Pressure relief valve may prevent effective ventilation in patients that require higher pressures.

14. Continuous positive airway pressure (CPAP)

    i. Used to improve ventilatory efficiency in spontaneously breathing patients in respiratory distress

    ii. Often used for patients with sleep apnea, has proven very effective for patients with COPD or pulmonary edema

    iii. Can help the patient avoid more invasive treatment such as intubation

    iv. Use of CPAP by EMTs based on local protocol

    v. Indications

        ➤ Conscious patients in moderate to severe respiratory distress

        ➤ Tachypnic patients with reduced respiratory efficiency

        ➤ Pulse oximetry is below 90%

    vi. Contraindications

➤ Apneic patients or patients unable to follow verbal commands

➤ Chest trauma, suspected pneumothorax, or patients with a tracheostomy

➤ Vomiting or suspected gastrointestinal bleeding

➤ Hypotension

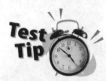

> *If you are undecided about ventilating your patient, then you probably should. If you're wrong, the patient will find a way to let you know. If you fail to ventilate a patient that needs it, the patient will continue to deteriorate.*

IV. SPECIAL SITUATIONS

A. Infants and Children

    1. Anatomical and physiological differences from adults

    i. The pediatric airway is more easily obstructed.

➤ The mouth and nose are smaller.

➤ The pediatric tongue is larger in proportion to the airway.

    ii. The pediatric head is larger in proportion to the body. Padding should be placed behind the shoulders in a supine patient to maintain alignment of the airway.

    iii. The lungs are smaller.

➤ Tidal volume provided during artificial ventilations is reduced.

➤ The risk of gastric distention, vomiting, and barotraumas is higher due to hyperventilation during artificial ventilations.

    iv. Hypoxia can develop much faster

➤ Infants and children have less oxygen reserves and a higher metabolic rate than adults.

➤ Bradycardia is common in pediatric patients experiencing significant hypoxia. Always assume a bradycardic infant or child is hypoxic and support oxygenation and ventilations aggressively.

    v.   Airway and respiratory problems are the primary cause of circulatory collapse.

  2. Signs of respiratory failure in pediatric patients

    i.   Bradycardia and poor muscle tone

    ii. Altered level of consciousness

    iii. Head bobbing, and grunting on exhalation

    iv. Seesaw breathing (chest and abdomen moving in opposition)

B. Ventilating Patients with a Tracheostomy Tube or Stoma

  1. The BVM will connect directly to a tracheostomy tube.

  2. To ventilate a patient with a stoma and no tracheostomy tube, use an infant or pediatric mask. Seal the mouth and nose during ventilation to prevent air escape. Release during exhalation.

  3. Tracheostomy tubes and stomas can become easily obstructed. If unable to ventilate effectively, suction the tube or stoma with a French suction catheter.

C. Foreign-body Airway Obstruction (FBAO)

    i.   The tongue is the number one cause of airway obstruction; however, foreign bodies such as vomit, food, latex balloons, and toys can also obstruct the airway.

    ii. Indications of complete or nearly complete FBAO

       ➤ Inability to cough, speak, or breath, or clutching the throat (conscious patient)

       ➤ Inability to artificially ventilate the patient despite repositioning airway and managing the tongue (unconscious patient)

    iii. Management of FBAO

       ➤ Conscious adults and children. Administer conscious abdominal thrusts until the obstruction is relieved or until the patient loses consciousness.

       ➤ Conscious infants. Administer a series of five back blows and five chest thrusts until the obstruction is relieved or until the patient loses consciousness.

> ➤ Unconscious patients (all ages)

— Initiate CPR.

— Before attempting ventilations, inspect the airway for visible foreign bodies. Remove if able.

D. Dentures

1. Dentures are often secured in place and can be left alone.

2. If dentures are loose, they should be removed.

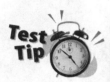

The test will likely include many scenario-based questions. These can be mentally taxing. Read each question carefully, looking for key terms and relevant information. National Registry scenario-based questions do not contain a lot of irrelevant information. The information provided in the question is important. Use the information to guide your answer. Avoid "looking for zebras"—which means don't let "what if" possibilities not included in the question unduly influence your answer.

Read the information provided by the NREMT related to the implementation of the 2010 AHA guidelines for CPR at the Resources link found at www.nremt.org.

PRACTICE QUESTIONS

1. Which of the following is the backup system to the CO_2 drive?

   A. carbon dioxide drive

   B. hypoxic drive

   C. anoxic drive

   D. oxygen drive

2. You have just initiated BVM ventilations for your apneic patient. Which of the following is most important to help determine if artificial ventilations are being delivered effectively?

   A. Check the pupillary response.

   B. Assess distal pulses.

   C. Auscultate lung sounds.

   D. Palpate the chest.

3. Which of the following indicates the need for supplemental oxygen by nasal cannula or non rebreather?

   A. An SaO_2 reading of 93%

   B. Clear bilateral lung sounds

   C. Slow and shallow respirations

   D. Warm, dry skin

4. Your patient is responsive only to painful stimuli. The airway is clear. How should you manage the patient's airway?

   A. Suction the airway.

   B. Insert an OPA.

   C. Insert an NPA.

   D. Begin artificial ventilations.

5. Due to the risk of hypoxia, suction time should not exceed

   A. 30 seconds for an adult.

   B. 30 seconds for a child.

   C. 15 seconds for an infant.

   D. 15 seconds for an adult.

ANSWERS

1. **B.**

   The hypoxic drive is the backup system to the CO_2 drive.

2. **C.**

   Two of the most important assessments to determine if artificial ventilations are being delivered effectively are auscultating lung sounds and observing for chest rise and fall.

3. **A.**

   An SaO_2 below 94% indicates the need for supplemental oxygen. Slow, shallow respirations indicate the need for artificial ventilations, not a nasal cannula or NRB. Clear lung sounds and warm, dry skin are normal findings.

4. **C.**

   The patient has a clear airway, so suction is not needed. The patient has a decreased LOC, so insertion of an NPA is indicated. The OPA is contraindicated because the patient is not unresponsive. The need for artificial ventilations is based on the patient's breathing status (not provided), not the patient's LOC.

5. **D.**

   Suctioning increases the risk of hypoxia. Suction time should not exceed 15 seconds for an adult, 10 seconds for pediatric patients, and 5 seconds for infants.

History Taking, Vital Signs, and Monitoring Devices

I. HISTORY TAKING

A. Chief Complaint

1. The chief complaint is the patient's primary reason for calling EMS.

2. The patient history will generally begin by determining the chief complaint.

3. If unable to determine the chief complaint from the patient, question family, bystanders, etc.

4. Other EMS providers can simultaneously begin other assessments or interventions as resources and the patient's condition allow.

B. History of Present Illness (HPI)

1. Once the chief complaint has been established, begin obtaining the history of present illness.

2. The HPI includes

    i. basic patient information, such as age, sex, and weight

    ii. additional information about the chief complaint

    iii. associated signs and symptoms

    iv. general health status

    v. past medical history (PMH), including medications and allergies

C. Techniques for History Taking

1. Notes. It is unlikely you will accurately remember all the information without taking notes.

2. Open-ended questions

   i.   Open-ended questions require the patient to respond with more than just "yes" or "no." These questions require a descriptive response.

   ii. When you want the patient to describe things in his or her own words, open-ended questions are preferred. Examples:

   ➤ "Why did you call for help today?"

   ➤ "How would you describe the pain?"

   ➤ "What were you doing when this started?"

   iii. Open-ended questions take longer to answer but provide more information from the patient's perspective.

3. Closed-ended questions

   i.   Closed-ended questions can be answered much faster and typically require only a "yes" or "no" response.

   ii. Closed-ended questions may be preferred when time is critical. For example, "Are you choking?" is more appropriate than "Can you describe how it feels to be choking?"

   iii. Closed-ended questions can also be useful if the patient is only able to speak short sentences due to severe pain or respiratory distress.

   iv. Closed-ended questions are faster but can lead the patient into answers that may be less accurate or insightful.

4. Active listening techniques

   i.   It is more effective to have one provider take responsibility for obtaining the patient history. If several providers are directing questions to the patient, it is harder to establish a rapport and keep the process organized.

   ii. Facilitate communication with your patient by facing him, maintaining eye contact, and providing verbal or nonverbal cues that you are listening.

   iii. Repeating what the patient has said demonstrates you are listening and may encourage the patient to provide more information.

   iv. Avoid interrupting the patient.

   v.   Attempt to clarify nonspecific statements.

   vi. Your questions should not be biased or judgmental.

vii. Showing empathy will help you establish a rapport with the patient. Example: "I can understand why you feel that way."

viii. Address contradictions or unclear information obtained during the history. For example, the patient states he has no medical history, but is on prescription medications. Sometimes patients will state they are allergic to a medication, but upon further questioning describe common side effects of the medication.

ix. Ask patients the most important questions first. This is an example of having an organized approach but allowing for flexibility. For example, questioning your trauma patient about possible neck pain should be done very early in the assessment. This is probably a lower priority for a medical patient without trauma.

5. Aids to history taking

  i. **SAMPLE** history

  ➤ **S**igns and symptoms

   — Signs are findings you can objectively see, feel, hear, or smell. Examples: vomiting, deformity, wheezing.

   — Symptoms are things the patient must tell you about. Examples: nausea, pain, dyspnea.

  ➤ **A**llergies

   — Any allergies, especially to prescription or over-the-counter medications.

  ➤ **M**edications

   — Any medications the patient takes regularly, including prescription, nonprescription medications, vitamins, and supplements

   — Any medications taken recently

   — Any illicit drugs

   — Any erectile dysfunction drugs

   — Spell the medications correctly, and write down the dose and frequency when possible.

   — Polypharmacy: many patients routinely take multiple medications.

  ➤ **P**ast pertinent history

   — Any relevant past medical history

— Cardiac, respiratory, diabetic, seizure, stroke history

— Any history similar to the current chief complaint

➤ **L**ast oral intake: most recent food and fluid intake

➤ **E**vents leading to incident

— What events led up to the current chief complaint?

— Anything unusual: activities, food, new medications, recent injury, etc.?

    ii. **OPQRST** is another memory aid to help obtain information about the patient's symptoms.

➤ *Note:* The OPQRST acronym is not a perfect fit for every chief complaint. There will be some complaints with essential questions not included in OPQRST. There will also be chief complaints when not every component of OPQRST is appropriate.

➤ This aid tends to work well with cardiac and respiratory patients and can be adapted to suit other chief complaints.

➤ **O**nset: "What were you doing when the symptoms began?"

➤ **P**rovocation: "Does anything make your symptoms better or worse?"

➤ **Q**uality: "How would you describe the pain?"

➤ **R**adiation: "Does the pain go anywhere?"

➤ **S**everity: "How would you rate the pain on a scale from 1 to 10, with 10 being the most severe?"

➤ **T**ime: "When did the symptom start?" *Note:* This is especially important with potential heart attack and stroke patients.

  6. Pertinent negatives

    i. Pertinent negatives are symptoms that are important to consider but are not present.

    ii. Those symptoms that are pertinent change depending on the patient's chief complaint. Examples might include

➤ determining if your trauma patient has neck pain

➤ determining if your chest pain patient has dyspnea

➤ determining if your patient lost consciousness

D. Special Situations

1. At times, it will be necessary to ask the patient about sensitive topics, such as assault, illicit drug use, use of erectile dysfunction medications, possible pregnancy, etc.

    i. Limit your questions to those that are relevant and necessary to care for your patient.

    ii. Be direct, but use a professional, nonjudgmental approach.

    iii. It may be helpful to question the patient with as much privacy as possible.

2. Some patient encounters can make it unusually challenging to obtain a patient history. Remember to utilize active-listening techniques and remain professional. Examples of challenging situations may include

    i. patients under the influence of alcohol or drugs

    ii. victims of sexual, physical, child, or elderly abuse or neglect

    iii. noncommunicative or overly talkative patients

    iv. patients with multiple complaints

    v. anxious, frightened, or emotional patients

    vi. patients with cognitive disabilities

    vii. non-English-speaking patients

    viii. patients with sensory challenges, such as hearing or sight impaired

    ix. patients with behavioral problems

    x. angry or hostile patients

II. VITAL SIGNS

Most vital signs provide a combination of quantitative (numerical) and qualitative (non-numerical) data. Every patient encounter should include at least two sets of vital signs. If unable to obtain at least two sets of vital signs, your patient care report should indicate why.

A. Baseline vital signs are the first set taken.

B. Trending is the comparison of vitals over time.

C. Frequency of Vital Signs

1. Stable patients: at least every 15 minutes

2. Unstable patients: at least every 5 minutes

D. The Standard Vital Signs

1. Respirations

2. Pulse

3. Blood pressure

4. Pupils

5. Skin

6. Pulse oximetry: the "sixth vital sign"

E. Respirations

1. Usually assessed by observing the patient's chest rise and fall. Sometimes easier to feel or auscultate respirations by placing a hand on the chest, or listening with a stethoscope.

2. Respiratory rate: the number of breaths per minute (bpm).

   i. Determined by counting the number of breaths (inhalations or exhalations, *not* both) for 30 seconds and doubling

   ii. Normal respiratory rates

   ➤ Adult: 12 to 20 bpm

   ➤ Children: 15 to 30 bpm

   ➤ Infants: 25 to 50 bpm

   iii. Abnormal respiratory rates

   ➤ Tachypnea: rapid breathing

   ➤ Bradypnea: slow breathing

3. Respiratory quality

   i. Rhythm and tidal volume of breathing

   ➤ Normal: regular rhythm and adequate chest rise and fall

   ➤ Shallow: minimal chest rise and fall

   ➤ Labored: increased work of breathing

   ➤ Irregular: abnormal breathing pattern

ii. Some consider auscultation of lung sounds part of the respiratory component of vital signs. Others consider lung sounds part of the physical exam. See chapter 9 for details on auscultation of lung sounds.

➤ Normal lung sounds are "clear and equal bilaterally."

➤ Abnormal lung sounds include absent, diminished, or unequal sounds, or wheezes or rales.

4. Sample documentation of respirations: "16 normal"

i. Always document both the quality and quantity of respirations.

F. Pulse

1. It is unlikely you will be able to palpate a pulse if the patient's blood pressure is below 60 mmHg systolic.

2. Location for pulse checks for patients that may be in cardiac arrest

i. Adults and children: carotid pulse

ii. Infants: brachial pulse

3. Location for pulse check for conscious patients

i. Adults and children: radial pulse

ii. Infants: brachial pulse

4. Pulse rate: the palpated one-minute pulse rate (cardiac contractions)

i. Determined by counting the number of pulses felt for 30 seconds and doubling. Irregular pulse rates may need to be counted for a full minute to be accurate.

ii. Normal pulse rates

➤ Adults: 60 to 100 beats per minute

➤ Children: about 80 to 120 beats per minute

➤ Infants: over 100 beats per minute

iii. Abnormal pulse rates

➤ Tachycardia: rapid pulse

➤ Bradycardia: slow pulse

5. Pulse quality and rhythm

   i.   Quality

      ➤ Strong

      ➤ Weak

   ii. Rhythm

      ➤ Regular

      ➤ Irregular

   iii. Sample documentation of pulse: "82 strong and regular"

G. Blood pressure (BP)

1. Blood pressure measures the pressure exerted against the walls of the arteries during contraction of the left ventricle and in between contractions.

2. Blood pressure is measured in millimeters of mercury (mmHg) with a sphygmomanometer (blood pressure cuff) and a stethoscope, or an automated noninvasive blood pressure monitoring device.

3. Sample blood pressure: 130/80

   i.   Systolic BP is the top number. Systole is the pressure exerted against the walls of the arteries during contraction.

   ii. Diastolic BP is the bottom number. Diastole is the pressure exerted against the walls of the arteries while the left ventricle is at rest.

   iii. Manual BP readings are always documented in even numbers.

4. Pulse pressure: the difference between the systolic and diastolic pressures

   i.   Normal pulse pressure: greater than 25% but less than 50% of systolic pressure

      ➤ Example: 130/80. 130 − 80 = 50.

   ii. Widened pulse pressure: pulse pressures above 50% of systolic

      ➤ Indicates possible head injury

      ➤ Example: 210/100

    iii. Narrow pulse pressure: pulse pressures below 25% of systolic

        ➤ Indicates possible hypoperfusion, tension pneumothorax, pericardial tamponade

        ➤ Example: 80/62

5. Normal blood pressures

    i. Normal blood pressures vary considerably, like height or weight.

    ii. Adults

        ➤ Estimating normal systolic pressure

           — Males: 100 + age (not to exceed 140 mmHg)

           — Females: 90 + age (not to exceed 130 mmHg)

        ➤ Estimating normal diastolic pressure

           — About 60 to 85 mmHg

        ➤ Examples

           — 35-year-old male: normal BP about 135 max/85 max

           — 20-year-old female: 110 max/85 max

           — 50-year-old male: 140 max/85 max

  iii. Children

        ➤ Estimating normal BP for ages 1 to 10 years

           — 80 + 2(age)/two-thirds systolic

        ➤ Example: 5-year-old patient: 90/60

        ➤ Hypotension

           — A systolic below 70 + 2(age) for ages 1 to 10 years

           — A pediatric patient with a blood pressure below 70 + 2(age) requires further evaluation for possible shock.

6. Abnormal blood pressures

    i. Hypertension: high blood pressure

    ii. Hypotension: low blood pressure

        ➤ Pediatric patients

           — A systolic BP below 70 + 2(age) is considered hypotension.

           — Example: A 5-year-old should *not* have a systolic BP below 80 mmHg.

7. Blood pressure by palpation

   i.   Palpation of a BP does not require a stethoscope.

   ii.   BP by palpation identifies the systolic BP only and is less accurate than auscultation.

   iii.   Always auscultate BP when able. Palpation should be used only when auscultation cannot be achieved.

   iv.   Palpating a systolic BP

      ➤ Inflate the BP cuff until the brachial pulse (distal to the cuff) or radial pulse can no longer be felt.

      ➤ Deflate the cuff slowly while feeling for the return of the brachial or radial pulse.

      ➤ Note the reading on the BP gauge when the pulse returns. This is the approximate systolic BP.

      ➤ Example documentation: 110/palp.

H. Orthostatic vital signs

1. Orthostatic vitals are an assessment of pulse and BP in two different positions, first supine and then standing. The second (standing) set should be taken after the patient has been standing for about two minutes.

2. Orthostatic vitals are used to assess for the possibility of hypovolemia. It is not a definitive diagnostic test but can be useful in certain circumstances.

3. Consult local protocol to determine if EMTs are permitted to perform this assessment.

4. Indication: suspected hypovolemia.

5. Contraindications

   i.   Suspected spinal injury

   ii.   Patients with altered or decreased level of consciousness

   iii.   Patients complaining of dizziness, weakness, or unable to stand

   iv.   Patients that are already significantly hypotensive prior to standing

   v.   Patients that are already known to be hypovolemic

      vi. If orthostatic assessment is not permitted per local protocol

  6. Orthostatically positive

      i. A positive orthostatic test is considered abnormal and indicates possible hypovolemia.

      ii. Positive orthostats requires both an increase in the heart rate of 10 to 20 beats per minute from supine to standing *and* a decrease in BP of 10 to 20 mmHg from seated to standing.

I. Pupils

  1. Pupils are assessed for size, equality, and reactivity.

  2. Size

      i. Size refers to pupil (dark center of the eye) size.

      ii. Look at pupil size in both eyes. Midsize = normal; dilated = large; constricted = small.

  3. Equality

      i. Equal: both pupils are round and equal size.

      ii. Unequal: pupils are of different size or shape.

  4. Reactivity

      i. Pupils should constrict (get smaller) when light is introduced and get larger in the dark. Note that pupils constrict, they don't "contract."

      ii. Pupillary constriction to light should be rapid, not sluggish.

      iii. Procedure

        ➤ Note pupil size before light is introduced.

        ➤ Using a penlight, shine the light into one pupil. Both should constrict.

        ➤ Repeat the procedure with the other eye.

      iv. Attempting to assess pupillary constriction with a penlight in a bright environment (outdoors, direct sun) will likely be ineffective.

      v. "Fixed and dilated": refers to pupils that are large and nonreactive to light. Indicates probability of severe illness or injury.

5. Documenting pupils. There are several ways to document pupils. Here are some examples:

   i. PEARL: pupils equal and reactive to light.

   ii. PERRL: pupils equal, round, reactive to light.

   iii. "Pupils midpoint, equal, reactive."

J. Skin

1. Four possible assessments for skin are color, temperature, condition, and capillary refill.

2. The skin provides clues to how well both the respiratory and the circulatory systems are functioning.

3. Skin color

   i. Check skin color by looking at the nail beds, palms of the hands, or soles of the feet. These areas should be pink for all complexions.

   ii. Abnormal skin color findings

      ➤ Pale: also called pallor; may indicate a lack of blood due to hypovolemia or vasoconstriction.

      ➤ Cyanotic: bluish color; may indicate a lack of oxygenated blood. Often appears in the nail beds or around the mouth first. A serious finding, but often a late finding.

      ➤ Flush: red skin; may indicate excessive heat, high temperature, exertion, or vasodilation.

      ➤ Jaundice: yellow skin; may indicate liver problems.

      ➤ Mottling: a "marbled" appearance to the skin combining cyanosis with other skin colors; may indicate shock or hypoperfusion.

4. Skin temperature

   i. Relative skin temperature

      ➤ Typically, EMTs assess the patient's relative (to touch) skin temperature, not a numerical reading with the use of a thermometer.

      ➤ Relative skin temperature is not exact, but it is quick and provides qualitative information about abnormally high or low temperatures.

➤ The EMT should spend a short time acclimating to the patient's environment before assessing relative skin temperature.

➤ Palpate the patient's skin near the core (back of the neck or upper back), not the forehead.

➤ Findings

— Warm: normal

— Cold: abnormal

— Hot: abnormal

ii. Normal body temperature. This temperature varies slightly based on location (oral, axillary, rectal); however, it is generally regarded as 98.6 degrees F or 37 degrees C.

5. Skin condition

i. Dry: normal

ii. Wet: abnormal

iii. Diaphoretic (excessive sweating): abnormal

iv. Clammy (cool and wet): abnormal

6. Capillary refill

i. Capillary refill is the time it takes for capillaries to refill with blood after being squeezed.

ii. Capillary refill is used to assess for possible hypoperfusion (shock).

iii. It is more reliable in infants and younger children. It is not considered reliable in older children or adults.

iv. The assessment is performed by compressing the nail bed or skin. This blanches (whitens) the area. Release and count the number of seconds it takes to return to normal color.

➤ Normal capillary refill in infants and younger children is two seconds or less.

➤ More than two seconds is considered "delayed" capillary refill and may indicate hypoperfusion.

➤ Delayed capillary refill alone is not enough to confirm hypoperfusion.

7. Sample documentation for skin: "skin warm, pink, dry, capillary refill less than 2 seconds"

III. MONITORING DEVICES

A. Pulse oximeter (see chapter 9)

B. Noninvasive Blood Pressure Monitoring

1. Automatically obtains a BP when manually activated or automatically at specified intervals

2. Frequently combined with other monitoring devices, such as a cardiac monitor/defibrillator

C. Glucometer

1. A glucometer (blood glucose meter) identifies the amount glucose in the blood.

2. Although not precise, glucometers provide reasonably accurate blood glucose levels for capillary and venous blood samples.

3. Unlike the other monitoring devices presented, glucometers are invasive (a blood sample is required) and they do not provide continuous monitoring.

4. In the United States, blood glucose levels are measured in mg/dL.

   i. Normal: 80 to 120 mg/dL

   ii. Hypoglycemia: 60 mg/dL or below

   iii. Hyperglycemia: over about 140 mg/dL

5. Indications

   i. Any patient with an altered or decreased level of consciousness

   ii. Any patient with a known or suspected diabetic history

6. Contraindications

   i. Not permitted per local protocol

   ii. Expired equipment or supplies

   iii. Equipment or supplies that have not passed quality control testing

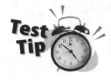

Test Tip

Good news! It is unlikely that you will see "all of the above" or "none of the above" as answer choices on the NREMT exam. Questions that include the word "except" are also rare.

PRACTICE QUESTIONS

1. While obtaining a patient history, you note the patient takes several prescription medications daily. This is known as

   A. multimeds.

   B. polypharmacy.

   C. unipharmacy.

   D. copharmacy.

2. Symptoms that are important to consider, but denied by the patient are known as

   A. pertinent negatives.

   B. chief complaints.

   C. dissociated symptoms.

   D. irrelevant assessments.

3. During your assessment, you note the patient has irregular breathing. This means the patient

   A. has an increased work of breathing.

   B. requires immediate ventilatory support.

   C. has minimal chest rise with each breath.

   D. presents with an abnormal breathing pattern.

4. Your 5-year-old patient is unresponsive. To determine if chest compressions are indicated, you should immediately assess the

   A. radial pulse.

   B. brachial pulse.

   C. carotid pulse.

   D. pedal pulse.

5. Your trauma patient has a widening pulse pressure. You should suspect

   A. a head injury.

   B. hypoperfusion.

   C. tension pneumothorax.

   D. pericardial tamponade.

ANSWERS

1. **B.**

   Simultaneous use of multiple medications by the same person is known as polypharmacy. The other options don't exist.

2. **A.**

   Pertinent negatives are symptoms that you should ask about, but are denied by the patient. Examples: a patient with chest pain that denies difficulty breathing, or a fall victim that denies neck pain.

3. **D.**

   Irregular breathing is an abnormal breathing pattern. The other options indicate labored breathing, inadequate breathing, and shallow breathing.

4. **C.**

   To determine if chest compressions are indicated for any patient over one year of age, you should assess the carotid pulse. For patients under one year of age, check the brachial pulse.

5. **A.**

   A widening pulse pressure indicates the possibility of a head injury with increased intracranial pressure. Hypoperfusion, tension pneumothorax, and pericardial tamponade will likely present with a narrowing pulse pressure.

Pharmacology

I. PHARMACOKINETICS AND PHARMACODYNAMICS

A. Pharmacokinetics is the study of how drugs enter the body, and are metabolized and eliminated.

B. Pharmacodynamics is the study of a drug's effects on the body.

II. THE "DRUG PROFILE"

A. The drug profile typically provides the most important information about the drug.

B. Health care providers who are permitted to administer drugs should know the drug profile for all drugs within their scope of practice.

C. Consult your medical direction or state EMS authority for an approved drug profile

D. Components of the drug profile should include the following:

1. Name

    i. Trade name: a brand name for a drug that has typically been trademarked by the manufacturer. Example: Nitro-Bid

    ii. Generic name: a name that is not trademarked and can be used by any manufacturer. Example: nitroglycerin

2. Class. The drug class identifies what "family" of medications the drug belongs to. Examples: anti-anginal, vasodilator

3. Mechanism of action (MOA)

   i. The MOA describes how the drug does what it does or its intended effects. Example: dilates blood vessels, increases myocardial oxygen supply

   ii. Drugs either stimulate or inhibit something the body is already capable of doing.

       ➤ Agonists: medications that stimulate an effect. Example: an asthmatic using an inhaler to increase bronchodilation

       ➤ Antagonists: medications that inhibit an effect. Example: taking aspirin to reduce pain

4. Indications. Situations in which the drug should be considered for administration. Example: chest pain

5. Contraindications

   i.   Situations in which the drug should not be given. Example: hypotension

   ii. Typically, if a patient meets both the indication and the contraindication criteria, the drug is *not* given.

   iii. Some drugs have "relative" contraindications that allow the provider some discretion. Usually, this occurs in situations where withholding the drug may be more harmful than administering the drug.

6. Dose and route of administration

   i. Dose: the amount of drug that should be given. Example: 0.4 mg

   ii. Route of administration: how the drug should be administered. Example: sublingual tablet or spray

       ➤ Enteral medications enter the body through the digestive system. Example: oral medications

       ➤ Parenteral medications enter the body through any means other than enteral. Examples: intramuscular and intravenous medications

7. Side effects. Any effects the drug may have other than those that are desired. Examples: hypotension, headache

8. Supply. The form in which the drug is supplied to the EMS provider. Example: nitroglycerin is supplied as tablets or spray, 0.4 mg per each tablet or spray

9. Special considerations. Any information unique to the drug that providers should be aware of. Example: nitroglycerin is heat and light sensitive and should be stored in a cool, dry place out of direct sunlight

III. ROUTES OF ADMINISTRATION

A. Enteral Route

1. Oral (PO): by mouth

   i. Slow onset of action, safe but unpredictable absorption.

   ii. Aspirin, activated charcoal, and oral glucose are all given orally.

B. Parenteral routes used by EMTs

1. Intramuscular (IM): directly into the muscle

   i. Rapid absorption, not quite as fast as intravenous (IV) or intraosseous (IO); faster than oral.

   ii. Less reliable absorption than IV or IO.

   iii. EpiPen is administered via intramuscular injection.

2. Inhalation: inhaled into the lungs

   i. Rapid onset.

   ii. Oxygen, metered-dose inhaler (MDI) medications, and small-volume nebulizer (SVN) medications are administered through inhalation.

3. Intranasal (IN): through the nose

   i. Intranasal drug administration provides a rapid onset of action and is an emerging method of drug administration in EMS.

   ii. IN medications are often delivered as a mist using a mucosal atomizer device (MAD)

   iii. Naloxone can be administered IN, and more IN medications are likely coming for EMS providers.

4. Sublingual (SL): under the tongue

   i. Faster onset than oral.

   ii. Nitroglycerin is administered SL.

IV. MEDICATION FORMS

A. Tablets or capsules: pill forms typically administered PO

B. Solutions: medication in liquid form; contains one or more substances that will not separate

C. Suspension: medication suspended in a liquid that easily separates or settles and must be mixed prior to administration

D. Metered dose inhaler (MDI) and small-volume nebulizer (SVN): medication in aerosolized form for inhalation

E. Gels: semiliquid medications, similar in consistency to toothpaste

F. Gas: medication in gas form, such as oxygen

V. ADMINISTERING MEDICATIONS

A. Medical Direction. EMTs must have online or offline medical direction to administer medications.

B. Patient History and Physical
   1. In most cases, it is important to complete a thorough history and physical prior to administering a medication.
   2. Determine what medications the patient takes regularly or has taken to treat the current complaint prior to your arrival.
   3. Complete the necessary physical exam, such as lung sounds, prior to administering a medication.
   4. Obtain vital signs prior to administering medications.

C. The "Six Rights" of Drug Administration
   1. Right patient. Make sure the drug is administered to the right patient.
   2. Right drug. Make sure the patient receives the correct drug.
   3. Right route. Make sure the drug is administered properly.
   4. Right amount. Make sure the patient receives the correct dose.

5. Right time. Make sure the patient receives the drug at the right time.

6. Right documentation. Make sure the PCR accurately documents the relevant information about the drug administration and response.

D. Second EMS Provider Confirmation. It is always a good idea to consult with another EMS provider on scene to confirm the safety and accuracy of any drug administration, dose, expiration date, etc.

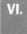 **VI. REASSESSMENT**

Following administration of a drug, reassess the chief complaint, vitals, and relevant history and physical exam.

 VII. MEDICATIONS CARRIED BY THE EMT

A. Consult local protocol; however, EMTs are typically permitted to carry

1. oxygen

2. oral glucose

3. aspirin

4. activated charcoal

5. epinephrine auto-injector pen

6. naloxone

B. Use of these drugs requires medical direction, either online or offline, per local protocol.

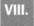 **VIII. MEDICATIONS *NOT* CARRIED BY THE EMT**

A. EMTs are *not* permitted to carry the following mediations but can assist the patient in taking them if they are prescribed to the patient and not expired:

1. MDI or SVN drugs for respiratory problems

2. Nitroglycerin

B. Use of these drugs requires medical direction, either online or offline, per local protocol.

IX. DRUG INFORMATION SOURCES

A. Medical direction and state EMS authorities

B. Package inserts (included with drug packaging)

C. Mobile device apps

D. Poison control centers: 1-800-222-1222 (U.S. only)

E. EMS drug reference guides

X. DRUG PROFILES

A. Activated Charcoal

1. Names: activated charcoal, Actidose, Super-Char, Liqui-Char

2. Class: adsorbent

3. Mechanism of action: adheres (binds) many drugs and chemicals, preventing their absorption from the gastrointestinal tract

4. Indication: recently ingested poisons

5. Contraindications

   i. Decreased level of consciousness

   ii. Inability to swallow

   iii. Ingestion of acids, alkalis, or hydrocarbons (See chapter 19 for information about caustics and hydrocarbons.)

   iv. Expired medication

   v. Lack of medical direction

6. Dose and route

   i. Adult dose is 1 gram per kilogram of body weight.

   ii. Pediatric dose is 25 to 50 grams.

   iii. Administered orally.

7. Side effects

    i.   Nausea and vomiting

    ii. Dark, tarry stool

8. Packaging: Supplied in 15-, 25-, or 50-gram bottles or tubes

9. Special considerations

    i.   Medication will settle. Shake before administering.

    ii. Use caution if you suspect the patient's level of consciousness may deteriorate.

    iii. Have suction ready.

    iv. Activated charcoal with Sorbitol should *not* be used on pediatric patients, hypovolemic patients, or dehydrated patients due to risk of severe diarrhea.

B. Aspirin

1. Names: acetylsalicylic acid, aspirin, Anacin, Bayer

2. Class: anti-inflammatory, anti-platelet aggregate, antipyretic

3. Mechanism of action: reduces inflammation, decreases platelet aggregation, reduces fever

4. Indication: chest pain

5. Contraindications

    i.   Allergy to medication

    ii.   Decreased level of consciousness

    iii. Inability to swallow

    iv.   Recent bleeding, active ulcer

    v.   Pediatric patient

    vi.   Expired medication

    vii. Lack of medical direction

6. Dose and route

    i.   160 to 325 mg (2 to 4 pediatric chewables)

    ii. Administered orally

7. Side effects

    i.   Nausea and vomiting

       ii.   Stomach pain

      iii. Bleeding

      iv. Allergic reaction

      v.   May lead to Reye's syndrome in pediatric patients

   8. Packaging: 81-mg pediatric chewables

C. MDI and SVN Medications

   1. Many drugs come in MDI form and are used to treat respiratory distress. It is not practical to learn them all. Focus on the most common. The drug profile for most others will be similar.

   2. Names

      i.   EMTs will typically help administer metered-dose inhaler (MDI) medications considered "rescue inhalers," not maintenance inhalers. Common rescue inhalers include

        ➤ albuterol, also knows as Proventil, Ventolin

        ➤ ipratropium bromide, also known as Atrovent

        ➤ isoetharine, also knows as Bronkosol

        ➤ Alupent, also known as Metaprel or metaproterenol

      ii. Small-volume nebulizers (SVN) aerosolize respiratory medications by connecting to an SVN machine or an oxygen source.

        ➤ Medication is added to the SVN and inhaled through a mouthpiece.

        ➤ Respiratory patients often have home SVN machines.

        ➤ Onset of action is rapid.

        ➤ SVNs can be easier to use than an MDI.

        ➤ The SVN base can be connected to a nonrebreather (NRB) mask with reservoir removed.

   3. Class: bronchodilator

   4. Mechanism of action: relaxes bronchial smooth muscle, improving air exchange

   5. Indications: dyspnea, asthma, reactive airway disease

   6. Contraindications

      i.   Allergy to medication

      ii.   Patient unable to follow commands

      iii. Expired medication

      iv. Medication not prescribed to patient

      v.   Lack of medical direction

7. Dose and route

      i.   One to two inhalations

      ii.   Inhaled

8. Side effects

      i.   Tachycardia

      ii.   Hypertension

      iii. Increased myocardial oxygen demand

      iv. Restlessness, anxiousness

9. Packaging: MDI

10. Special considerations

      i.   Successful administration requires cooperation and coordination between patient and EMT.

      ii.   Some patients may have a spacer device to simplify administration.

D. Epi Auto-Injector

1. Names: Epinephrine, EpiPen, Epi auto-injector, Adrenaclick

2. Class: sympathomimetic, bronchodilator

3. Mechanism of action: peripheral vasoconstriction, increased heart rate, bronchodilation

4. Indication: anaphylaxis

5. Contraindications

      i.   Expired medication

      ii.   Lack of medical direction

6. Dose and route

      i.   One auto injector

      ii.   Administered IM, usually lateral mid-thigh

7. Side effects

    i. Tachycardia

    ii. Hypertension

    iii. Increased myocardial oxygen demand

    iv. Restlessness, anxiousness

8. Packaging: Auto-injector; adult and pediatric auto-injectors available.

9. Special considerations

    i. Must be administered rapidly for severe, life-threatening allergic reactions.

    ii. Needle will go through clothing if necessary.

    iii. Must hold in place for several seconds to allow medication to enter patient.

    iv. Dispose of sharps properly immediately after administration.

E. Naloxone

1. Names: naloxone, Narcan, Narcan Nasal Spray

2. Class: narcotic antagonist

3. Mechanism of action: reverses effects of opioid (narcotic) medications, such as respiratory depression and decreased LOC

4. Indication: suspected opioid (narcotic) overdose

5. Contraindications

    i. Allergy to medication

    ii. Expired medication

    iii. Lack of medical direction

6. Dose and route

    i. Adult dose is 1 mg each nostril with spray or liquid in syringe using a mucosal atomizer device (MAD). Can be repeated as necessary with medical direction approval.

    iii. Administered intranasally.

7. Side effects

    i. Possible combative behavior

    ii. Possible withdrawal symptoms in narcotic dependent patients

8. Packaging: liquid (usually 1 mg per mL) or spray bottle

9. Special considerations

    i. Additional doses may be needed for continued effects

    ii. Be prepared for possible combative patient and vomiting.

F. Nitroglycerin

1. Names: nitroglycerin, Nitrostat, Nitrobid, Nitrolingual

2. Class: antianginal, vasodilator

3. Mechanism of action: vasodilation, decreased myocardial oxygen demand, increased myocardial oxygen supply

4. Indications: Chest pain, suspected angina or myocardial infarction

5. Contraindications

    i. Expired medication

    ii. Not prescribed to patient

    iii. Hypotension

    iv. Recent use of Viagra, Cialis, Levitra, or another erectile dysfunction medication

    v. Head injury

    vi. Lack of medical direction

6. Dose and route

    i. 0.4 mg sublingual

    ii. Spray or tablet

7. Side effects

    i. Reflex tachycardia

    ii. Hypotension

    iii. Headache

    iv. Burning under the tongue

    v. Nausea, vomiting

8. Packaging: 0.4 mg per dose tablets or spray

G. Oral Glucose

  1. Names: oral glucose, Glutose, Insta-Glucose

  2. Class: oral hyperglycemic

  3. Mechanism of action: increases blood glucose level

  4. Indication: hypoglycemia

  5. Contraindications

     i.   Decreased level of consciousness

     ii. Inability to swallow

     iii. Expired medication

     iv. Lack of medical direction

  6. Dose and route

     i.   Half a tube to one tube

     ii. Administered orally

  7. Side effects: Nausea and vomiting

  8. Packaging: Tube containing about 15 to 25 grams of oral glucose

H. Oxygen

  1. Names: oxygen

  2. Class: inhaled gas

  3. Mechanism of action: increases oxygen concentration

  4. Indication: suspected hypoxia

  5. Contraindication: unsafe environment

  6. Dose and route

     i.   Preferred route: 15 lpm via nonrebreather mask

     ii. Inhaled

  7. Side effects: rare respiratory depression with COPD patients

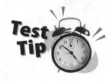

The NREMT certification exam ends for one of three reasons:

1. Most often, the test ends because the candidate has passed (you!) or failed (not you!) the exam.

2. It is a timed test. For EMT candidates, the time limit is two hours. The computer continuously notifies candidates about how much time remains.

3. Because the test is constantly adapting to you, the number of questions varies. EMT candidates will face a minimum of about 70 and a maximum of 120 questions.

PRACTICE QUESTIONS

1. Which of the following medications is administered enterally?

   A. EpiPen

   B. Nitroglycerin

   C. Oral glucose

   D. Naloxone

2. Which of the following medications is used to reverse the effects of an opioid overdose?

   A. Narcan

   B. Epinephrine

   C. Glucagon

   D. Albuterol

3. Which of the following is a common side effect of nitroglycerin administration?

   A. Reduced heart rate

   B. Elevated blood pressure

   C. Decreased chest pain

   D. Reduced blood pressure

4. EMTs can help administer, but cannot carry, which of the following medications?

   A. MDI

   B. Oral glucose

   C. Oxygen

   D. Aspirin

5. Which of the following medications is an adsorbent?

   A. Oral glucose

   B. Activated charcoal

   C. Epinephrine

   D. Naloxone

ANSWERS

1. **C.**

   Enteral medications enter the body through the digestive system and include activated charcoal, aspirin, and oral glucose.

2. **A.**

   Narcan (naloxone) is a narcotic antagonist used to reverse the effects of an opioid (narcotic) overdose.

3. **D.**

   Common side effects of nitroglycerin administration include hypotension, headache, burning under the tongue, and sometimes tachycardia. Decreased chest pain is a desired effect, not a side effect.

4. **A.**

   EMTs do not carry MDI medications or nitroglycerin.

5. **B.**

   Activated charcoal is an adsorbent. Oral glucose is a hyperglycemic agent. Epinephrine is a sympathomimetic. Naloxone is a narcotic antagonist.

Patient Assessment

I. THE EMT APPROACH TO PATIENT ASSESSMENT

A. Five Components of Patient Assessment

1. Scene size-up

2. Primary assessment

3. Patient history

4. Secondary assessment

5. Reassessment

B. The scene size-up always comes first, and doesn't end until the call ends. The primary assessment always follows the scene size-up and precedes all other components of patient assessment. The order and priority of the patient history and secondary assessment can change based on the patient's complaint and condition.

1. Significant trauma patients tend to demand a more intensive primary and secondary assessment than other types of patients. For significant trauma patients, the secondary assessment would typically be a higher priority than the patient history.

2. Conscious medical patients often demand a more thorough patient history than trauma patients. For these patients, the patient history would typically be a higher priority than the secondary assessment.

3. The NREMT skill sheets for patient assessment trauma and patient assessment medical hint at the above concepts. Look at how many points are awarded for the secondary assessment and the patient history on both skill sheets.

C. Regardless of the patient's condition, the patient assessment must be organized and methodical.

II. THE SCENE SIZE-UP

A. The scene size-up begins as soon as the call is received, and does not end until patient care is transferred and the call is ended.

B. Components of Scene Size-Up

1. Scene safety

    i. Your safety is the first priority. If the scene is safe, continue with your assessment. If the scene is not safe and you can make it safe very quickly, do so. If not, leave immediately and request assistance.

    ii. EMS personnel are required to wear a National Standards Institute 207 certified safety vest at all accident scenes or anytime working near traffic.

    iii. A portable, durable, high-intensity flashlight should be carried at all times.

    iv. Keep a portable radio and cell phone with you when possible.

    v. Position emergency vehicle for easy access, and use as a traffic barrier when needed.

    vi. Staging. Some EMS systems will dispatch the EMS crew to a scene that has not been secured by law enforcement, but will be told to "stage." Staging allows the EMS crew to respond to the call but remain a safe distance away until cleared by law enforcement.

2. Standard precautions. Take standard precautions and appropriate personal protective equipment (PPE). (Review chapter 3 for additional information on standard precautions.)

3. Number of patients/additional resources

    i. Determine the number of patients.

    ii. Request additional resources as needed, such as advanced life support, transport, or extrication.

4. Mechanism of injury (MOI)/Nature of illness (NOI)

    i. The patient is usually the best source of information for MOI and NOI; however, at times it will be necessary to question family or bystanders.

   ii. Mechanism of injury (trauma patients)

> ➤ Determine how the injury occurred. Examples: fall injury, motor vehicle accident, assault.

— Blunt trauma: an injury that does not penetrate the skin

— Penetrating trauma: an injury that penetrates the skin

> ➤ Understanding the MOI can help predict injuries, make treatment decisions, and select appropriate hospital destinations.

   iii. Nature of illness (medical patients)

> ➤ Determine the nature of the patient's medical complaint.

> ➤ NOI will be related to the chief complaint, but is not the same thing. For example, the patient could have a chief complaint of chest pain, but it could be the result of trauma. This would require an assessment of the MOI, not the NOI.

III. PRIMARY ASSESSMENT

A. The primary assessment begins when you arrive at the patient.

B. The purpose of the primary assessment is to identify and treat immediately life-threatening conditions.

C. Manual cervical spine stabilization. If cervical spine (c-spine) injury is suspected, manual c-spine precautions should be taken immediately according to local protocol.

D. General Impression

1. The general impression is the information you are able to immediately determine upon arriving at the patient, such as the patient's age, sex, level of distress, and overall appearance.

2. Determine level of patient exposure needed. At times, it will be necessary to remove some or all of the patient's clothing to assess for life-threatening conditions. If exposure is indicated, protect the patient's privacy as best you can.

E. Position Patient

   1. If the patient is prone, log roll the patient to the supine position.

   2. Move the patient with manual c-spine precautions if indicated.

F. Level of Consciousness

   1. During the primary assessment, the first assessment of level of consciousness (LOC) is general, not specific. Determine if the patient is

      i. conscious and alert

      ii. conscious and altered

      iii. unconscious

   2. AVPU scale. The **AVPU** scale can be used to rapidly determine the patient's general responsiveness.

      i. **A** = awake and alert

      ii. **V** = responsive to voice

      iii. **P** = responsive to pain

      iv. **U** = unresponsive

   3. Note for unresponsive patients: The 2010 guidelines for emergency cardiac care and basic life support advocate checking for cardiac arrest and initiating CPR as quickly as possible. To accomplish this, a **CAB** approach to assessment is recommended for unresponsive patients.

      i. Circulation. If the patient is unresponsive, with no signs of breathing, or agonal breaths, and no confirmed pulse within 10 seconds, initiate CPR and incorporate the automated external defibrillator (AED) as soon as it is available. CPR should begin with compressions, not ventilations.

      ii. Airway. Check airway and intervene as needed. Opening the airway in unresponsive patients should be done after determining the need for chest compressions.

      iii. Breathing. Assess breathing and intervene as needed. Assessing for breathing (look, listen, feel) and artificial ventilations are performed after determining the need for chest compressions.

4. Person, place, time, and event. If the patient is awake and alert, a more thorough assessment of LOC should be completed.

   i.   Person. The patient knows his or her name.

   ii. Place. The patient knows where he or she is.

   iii. Time. The patient knows the year, month, and approximate date and time.

   iv. Event. The patient can describe the MOI or NOI.

G. Airway

   1. Assess the airway and intervene as needed.

   2. The patient's LOC is a key factor in determining what airway interventions are needed. Do not assume patients with a decreased LOC are capable of protecting their own airway.

   3. Airway assessments and interventions should be performed in the following order:

      i.   Manual airway maneuvers as needed

           ➤ Head-tilt, chin-lift if no spinal injury suspected

           ➤ Jaw thrust maneuver if spinal injury suspected

      ii. Suction as needed

      iii. Mechanical airway adjuncts as needed

           ➤ Oropharyngeal airway (OPA) for unresponsive patients

           ➤ Consider nasopharyngeal airway (NPA) for patients with decreased LOC (See chapter 9 for additional information on airway management.)

H. Breathing

   1. Assess respiratory rate, quality, and auscultate lung sounds.

   2. Provide supplemental oxygen or artificial ventilations as needed.

   3. Manage life-threatening conditions associated with breathing. Examples:

      i.   Flail chest: initiate artificial ventilations.

      ii. Sucking chest wound: apply an occlusive dressing.

I. Circulation

1. Assess central versus peripheral pulses.

   i.   Initiate CPR as needed.

   ii.   Check the brachial pulse on infants.

2. Assess for and control life-threatening bleeding.

   i.   Direct pressure is the first technique to control external bleeding.

   ii.   *Note:* Any life-threatening bleeding on the posterior must also be controlled during the primary assessment.

3. Check skin color.

4. Check capillary refill for pediatric patients. (See chapter 9 for additional information on breathing.)

J. *Note:* The posterior should be assessed for life-threatening conditions during the primary assessment. Conditions such as a sucking chest wound or life-threatening bleeding should be found and managed before the primary assessment is completed.

K. Rapid Scan

1. Perform a rapid scan to identify any remaining life-threatening, such as signs of internal bleeding, unstable pelvis, closed femur fractures.

2. The rapid scan exists specifically to identify any remaining life threats and should take no longer than 90 seconds. Do *not* spend time on non-life-threatening conditions during the rapid scan.

3. The rapid scan should include inspection, palpation, and auscultation as needed.

   i.   Some conditions can only be seen or felt, not both.

   ii.   Auscultate lung sounds here if not done during breathing or if there is a change in the patient's condition or bag compliance.

L. Transport Priority

1. Determine if the patient should be transported rapidly, or if the patient's condition allows continued care on scene.

2. The Golden Period. This period starts when the injury occurs and does not end until the patient receives definitive care.

    i. Survival rates from shock and serious trauma diminish if the patient does not receive definitive care rapidly after the injury.

    ii. The Platinum 10 Minutes. This is critical for patients with significant trauma or who are showing signs of shock.

> ➤ The goal should be to assess the patient, manage life-threatening conditions, package the patient for transport, and begin transport within 10 minutes.

> ➤ Do *not* delay transport of a high-priority patient to manage non-life-threatening conditions.

IV. PATIENT HISTORY

A. Identify the chief complaint.

B. Obtain SAMPLE history. (See chapter 10 for additional information.)

C. Assess for associated symptoms and pertinent negatives relative to the mechanism of injury or nature of illness.

V. SECONDARY ASSESSMENT

A. The secondary assessment should *not* delay patient transport.

B. The secondary assessment is designed to identify any remaining signs, conditions, or injuries.

C. All potentially life-threatening conditions should already be managed.

D. The secondary assessment can be a complete head-to-toe assessment or a focused exam that assesses only relevant areas.

1. The secondary assessment should include inspection, palpation, and auscultation as needed.

2. Head-to-toe assessment should be performed when the patient

    i. is unresponsive or otherwise unable to provide feedback

    ii. has experienced multisystem trauma

    iii. is a high transport priority

3. Format for head-to-toe assessment

    i. Head and neck

       ➤ Palpate and inspect for DCAP-BTLS.

           — DCAP-BTLS is an acronym used to help remember many of the things that should be assessed during the head-to-toe assessment: **D**eformities, **C**ontusions, **A**brasions, **P**enetrating injuries, **B**urns, **T**enderness, **L**acerations, **S**welling.

        ➤ Assess pupils.

        ➤ Assess ears for drainage and behind the ears for bruising.

        ➤ Assess the neck for pain, tenderness and JVD.

    ii. Chest

        ➤ Assess for DCAP-BTLS.

        ➤ Assess for equal rise and fall; auscultate lung sounds.

        ➤ Assess for medication patches and medical devices.

    iii. Abdomen

        ➤ Assess for DCAP-BTLS.

        ➤ Assess for rigidity, distention.

    iv. Pelvis

        ➤ Assess for DCAP-BTLS.

        ➤ Assess for instability and crepitus.

        ➤ Assess for incontinence.

        ➤ Do *not* palpate the pelvis if the patient already complains of pain.

    v. Extremities

        ➤ Assess distal pulse, motor, and sensation in all four extremities.

        ➤ Pulse: palpate for the presence of radial and dorsalis pedis pulses.

        ➤ Motor function: assess patient's ability to grip, push, and pull on command.

➤ Sensation: assess patient's ability to feel you palpate his fingers and toes.

➤ Check for medic alert tags or bracelets.

 vi. Posterior

➤ Assess the posterior for DCAP-BTLS.

➤ Auscultate posterior lung sounds.

 vii. *Note:* It is not necessary or appropriate to conduct a complete head-to-toe secondary assessment on every patient.

4. A focused exam can be considered when an alert patient has an isolated injury or has a specific medical complaint.

 i. During a focused exam, the EMT determines what areas are relevant and assesses only those areas.

 ii. The recommended components of a focused exam will vary based on the patient's condition, but lung sounds should be assessed on every patient if not already completed.

E. Baseline Vitals

1. Assess vitals, pulse oximeter, and blood glucose.

2. Repeat vitals as needed.

 i. Stable patient: at least every 15 minutes

 ii. Unstable patient: at least every 5 minutes

VI.   REASSESSMENT

A. The purpose of the reassessment phase is to monitor for changes in the patient's condition.

B. Complete reassessment at least every 5 minutes for unstable patients and every 15 minutes for stable patients.

C. Components of Reassessment

1. Reassess LOC, airway, breathing, and circulation.

2. Reassess chief complaint, interventions, and vitals.

D. The reassessment phase does not end until patient care is transferred; however, it can be interrupted if you discover something that requires immediate attention.

V. SUMMARY OF PATIENT ASSESSMENT

A. Scene Size-Up

1. Assess scene safety and take standard precautions.

2. Determine number of patients and need for additional resources.

3. Consider MOI or NOI.

B. Primary Assessment

1. Assess and manage ABCs (circulation first if patient unresponsive). Remember to check the posterior for life-threatening conditions as needed.

    i. Enact simultaneous manual c-spine precautions if needed.

    ii. Administer oxygen and ventilate as needed (SaO_2 of at least 94%).

2. Perform rapid scan as needed.

3. Determine transport priority.

C. Patient History

1. Take SAMPLE history.

D. Secondary Assessment

1. Perform head-to-toe assessment or focused exam as needed.

2. Assess vitals, lung sounds, pulse oximetry, blood glucose as needed.

E. Reassess

1. Monitor patient's airway, breathing, and circulatory status.

2. Repeat vitals and reassess interventions.

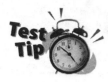

There are five assessment categories on the NREMT exam (see Chapter 1). Although patient assessment is not a specific category, it will be an integral part of the overall test content. A strong knowledge of patient assessment is essential to passing the certification exam.

Candidates should be thoroughly familiar with the NREMT patient assessment skill sheets prior to taking the certification exam. Memorize both as they will likely guide you to the correct answers on several questions during your certification exam!

PRACTICE QUESTIONS

1. You have completed the primary assessment on an unresponsive multi-system trauma patient. Which of the following should be done next?

   A. Obtain a patient history.

   B. Manage any secondary injuries.

   C. Assess baseline vital signs.

   D. Document your findings and interventions.

2. Which of the following statements regarding the primary assessment is correct?

   A. The primary assessment always precedes the patient history.

   B. The primary assessment is not necessary for conscious non-trauma patients.

   C. The primary assessment may follow the patient history for medical patients.

   D. The primary assessment should never take longer than 90 seconds.

3. You have completed the primary assessment on a conscious patient complaining of dyspnea. There is no trauma. Which of the following should be done next?

   A. Obtain a patient history.

   B. Manage any secondary injuries.

   C. Perform a detailed physical exam.

   D. Check the posterior for any injuries.

4. Which of the following is always your first priority while performing a physical exam on a patient?

   A. Identify and manage life-threatening conditions.

   B. Initiate transport within 10 minutes.

   C. You and your partner's safety.

   D. Requesting additional resources as needed.

5. What is the purpose of the rapid scan?

   A. Assess and manage the ABCs.

   B. Identify all secondary injuries.

   C. Reassess all injuries and interventions.

   D. Identify any remaining life-threats.

ANSWERS

1. C.

   For a multi-system trauma patient, the secondary assessment (including baseline vitals) would be a higher priority than the patient history, secondary injuries, or documentation.

2. A.

   The primary assessment must be completed on every patient and always precedes the patient history and secondary assessment. The time spent on the primary assessment is dictated by the patient's condition.

3. **A.**

   For a conscious non-trauma patient, the patient history is the best choice. The other choices are either not appropriate for this patient, or a lower priority than the patient history.

4. **C.**

   Your safety is always your first priority.

5. **D.**

   The rapid scan is completed after assessment and management of the ABCs and is specifically meant to identify any remaining life-threats.

PART IV

SHOCK, RESUSCITATION, AND MEDICAL EMERGENCIES

Chapter 3

Shock, Resuscitation, and AED

SHOCK

A. Pathophysiology of Shock

1. Perfusion is the adequate circulation of oxygenated blood throughout the body. Adequate perfusion is necessary to maintain homeostasis.

2. Shock, or hypoperfusion, is inadequate tissue perfusion. The cells of the body do not get the oxygen and nutrients they need from the circulatory system.

   i. Compensated shock: the early stage of shock. The body is still able to compensate for the hypovolemic state through defense mechanisms, such as increased heart rate and peripheral vasoconstriction.

   ii. Decompensated shock: late or "progressive" shock. The body can no longer compensate for the hypovolemic state, and blood pressure starts to fall.

   iii. Irreversible shock: final stage of shock. The patient will not survive once entering irreversible shock.

3. Figure 13-1 shows how shock can continue to spiral downward until death if not managed appropriately before it's too late.

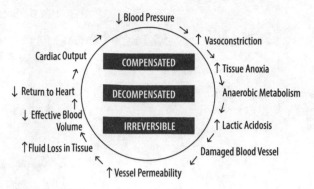

Figure 13-1: Shock Cycle

B. Three Primary Causes of Shock

1. Pump (heart) problems.
   Examples: myocardial infarction, cardiac trauma

2. Pipe (blood vessel) problems.
   Examples: anaphylaxis, spinal trauma, infection

3. Fluid (blood volume) problems.
   Examples: bleeding, vomiting, diarrhea

C. Compensation Mechanisms. The body will fight to protect itself during shock as long as possible.

1. Tachycardia. If there is a loss of circulating blood volume, the body will increase heart rate and cardiac force of contraction to compensate.

2. Peripheral vasoconstriction. The body will constrict peripheral blood vessels to try and increase blood pressure and increase perfusion to vital organs.

3. The body will increase the respiratory rate to improve oxygenation.

4. Falling blood pressure is a *late* sign of shock. It indicates the body's defense mechanisms are no longer working.

   i.   Assume any patient with suspected shock and hypotension is in decompensated shock. Treat as a high transport priority.

   ii. Pediatric patients can maintain their blood pressure until about half of their blood volume has been lost. Do *not* wait for hypotension to begin treating a pediatric patient for shock.

Signs of shock with hypotension in the pediatric population are ominous.

D. Types of Shock

1. Cardiogenic shock

   i. Cardiogenic shock is a pump problem.

   ii. The heart muscle cannot pump effectively, causing a backup of fluid, pulmonary edema, and hypotension.

      ➤ Pulmonary edema: accumulation of fluid in the lungs.

      ➤ Cardiogenic shock is caused by low cardiac output due to reduced preload, high afterload, or poor myocardial contractility.

   iii. Signs and symptoms of cardiogenic shock include hypotension, probable cardiac history, chest pain, respiratory distress, pulmonary edema, and altered level of consciousness (LOC).

2. Obstructive shock. This type of shock is a pump problem caused by mechanical obstruction of the heart muscle.

   i. Cardiac tamponade

      ➤ Fluid accumulates within the pericardial sac and compresses the heart. Also called pericardial tamponade.

      ➤ Signs and symptoms may include

         — jugular venous distention (JVD): filling of jugular veins in the neck

         — narrowing pulse pressures: systolic and diastolic pressures moving closer together

         — hypotension

   ii. Tension pneumothorax

      ➤ Air enters the chest cavity due to lung injury or sucking chest wound. Accumulating pressure compresses the lungs and great vessels.

      ➤ Signs and symptoms may include JVD, respiratory distress, diminished or absent lung sounds, poor compliance during artificial ventilations with bag valve mask (BVM), and tracheal deviation toward the unaffected side. Tracheal deviation is a very late sign.

3. Distributive shock

    i.   Distributive shock is a pipe (blood vessel) problem.

    ii.   It occurs due to widespread vasodilation, which causes blood pooling and relative hypovolemia.

       ➤ Relative hypovolemia: low volume relative to the size of the vascular space. Distributive shock expands blood vessels, making the vascular space bigger and the volume inadequate for effective circulation.

    iii. Anaphylactic shock (also known as anaphylaxis)

       ➤ A life-threatening form of severe allergic reaction due to three factors:

          — Massive vasodilation

          — Widespread vessel permeability (fluid leakage)

          — Bronchoconstriction

       ➤ Causes include medications, foods, bites, stings, environmental allergens.

       ➤ Signs and symptoms may include the following:

          — Skin: hives, swelling, itching, flushed or cyanotic color

          — Cardiovascular: weak pulses, hypotension

          — Respiratory: severe dyspnea, wheezing, respiratory failure

    iv. Neurogenic shock/spinal cord injury

       ➤ Neurogenic shock is caused by spinal cord damage, typically in the cervical region.

       ➤ It leads to massive, systemic vasodilation below the level of injury.

       ➤ Relative hypovolemia results due to dramatic increase in vascular space.

       ➤ Neurogenic shock interrupts the normal communication pathways between the central nervous system and the peripheral nervous system. This interferes with the body's normal compensatory mechanisms.

➤ Signs and symptoms may include the following:

— Mechanism of injury indicative of cervical-spine injury

— Hypotension

— Warm skin, normal color

   a. This is unusual because the skin is normally pale and cool during shock due to increased peripheral vasoconstriction.

   b. During neurogenic shock, the nervous system cannot stimulate peripheral vasoconstriction due to spinal cord injury.

— Heart rate that is *not* tachycardic

   a. This is unusual because the heart rate normally increases during shock to compensate for hypovolemia.

   b. During neurogenic shock, the nervous system cannot stimulate tachycardia due to spinal cord injury.

— Paralysis: Depending on the severity and location of injury, paralysis may impact the lower extremities, all extremities, and even the diaphragm.

— Respiratory paralysis

— Priapism: persistent, painful penile erection

i. Septic shock

➤ Septic shock is caused by severe infection, which damages blood vessels and increases plasma loss out of the vascular space.

➤ Blood vessels do not constrict well during septic shock, diminishing the body's ability to compensate.

➤ Although primarily a pipe (vessel) problem, septic shock also leads to hypovolemia due to vessel permeability, fever, increased respiratory rate, and often poor fluid intake while ill.

➤ Signs and symptoms of septic shock may include

— fever, chills, weakness

— recent illness, infection, or surgery

— altered level of consciousness, increased respiratory rate

— tachycardia, hypotension, pale, cool skin

— weak peripheral pulses and loss of appetite

  vi. Psychogenic shock

➤ Psychogenic shock is a pseudo-shock caused by sudden, temporary vasodilation that leads to syncope (fainting). Psychogenic shock does not typically present a problem because there is not sustained inadequate tissue perfusion.

➤ The sudden vasodilation interrupts blood flow to the brain, leading to a syncopal episode.

➤ Note that there are many causes of syncope, some serious. Psychogenic shock is only one of them.

4. Hypovolemic shock

  i. Hypovolemic shock is a fluid problem.

  ii. Hemorrhagic shock is a form of hypovolemic shock due to loss of whole blood. Note: hemorrhagic shock is always hypovolemic, but not all hypovolemia is due to hemorrhage.

  iii. Dehydration due to vomiting, diarrhea, or burns can also lead to hypovolemic shock.

  iv. Hypovolemic shock due to dehydration is common in pediatric and geriatric patients.

  v. Signs and symptoms of hypovolemic shock may include

➤ trauma, blunt or penetrating

➤ bleeding, altered LOC, nausea, vomiting, diarrhea

➤ tachycardia, pale, cool skin

➤ weak peripheral pulses, hypotension

E. Signs and Symptoms of Shock

1. Early signs and symptoms

  i. Many of the early signs and symptoms of shock are indications the body is attempting to protect itself.

      ii. Altered LOC

        ➤ Examples: restlessness, anxiousness, irritability

        ➤ An indication of early hypoxia

     iii. Tachycardia

     iv. Pale, cool skin: due to increased peripheral vasoconstriction

     v. Weak peripheral pulses: due to increased peripheral vasoconstriction

     vi. Increased respiratory rate

     vii. Thirst

     viii. Delayed capillary refill (over two seconds) in pediatric patients

2. Late signs and symptoms

     i.   Falling blood pressure

     ii. Irregular breathing

     iii. Mottling or cyanosis

     iv. Absent peripheral pulses

3. Remember, the presentation of neurogenic shock is unique due to the interruption in communication between the central and peripheral nervous systems.

     i.   Skin is typically warm, and heart rate is often normal.

     ii. Paralysis, including respiratory paralysis, could be immediate.

F. Managing Shock (See summary of assessment in chapter 12.)

1. Control bleeding.

2. Place the patient supine when possible. *Note:* Often those in cardiogenic or obstructive shock will not tolerate being placed supine.

3. Prevent loss of body heat.

4. Initiate rapid transport to appropriate facility. Remember the "Platinum 10 Minutes."

5. *Note:* There is no clear evidence that use of the pneumatic anti-shock garment (PASG) is beneficial for treating shock. Consult local protocol. If used, the PASG should *not* delay patient transport. (See chapter 23 for additional information on the PASG.)

II. RESUSCITATION

A. CPR Standards and Requirements

1. Candidates for NREMT certification must have a current and valid CPR credential equivalent to the American Heart Association's (AHA) Basic Life Support (BLS).

2. The NREMT certification exam for EMTs will reflect the current AHA guidelines.

3. The 2015 AHA BLS Provider Manual provides the standards for cardiopulmonary resuscitation that will be included on the NREMT exam.

4. For additional information about the 2015 AHA CPR Guidelines, visit *https://eccguidelines.heart.org/index.php/circulation/cpr-ecc-guidelines-2/*.

    i. *Note:* There may be other publications equivalent to the current AHA guidelines for CPR. Contact the NREMT (*www.nremt.org*) to determine what is considered equivalent to the AHA's BLS certification.

B. Highlights of 2015 Basic Life Support Guidelines

1. Emphasis is on high-quality compressions

    i. Rate of compression: 100-120 per minute

    ii. Depth of compression

    ➤ At least 2 inches (5 cm) for adults, but not more than 2.4 inches (6 cm)

    ➤ At least 1/3 depth of chest for infants and pediatric patients

    — About 2 inches for pediatric patients

    — About 1½ inches for infants

    iii. Allow full chest recoil between compressions

    iv. Minimum interruption in chest compressions

    ➤ Minimize interruption in chest compressions before and after shock with automatic external defibrillator (AED), when switching compressors, etc.

     v.   Compression to ventilation ratio

        ➤ Single rescuer (any age): 30:2

        ➤ Two rescuers with infants and children: 15:2

2. CAB sequence, not ABC sequence, is used for unresponsive patients

    i.   Circulation first, then airway and breathing

    ii. Do not delay checking a pulse or initiating chest compressions to look, listen, and feel for respirations.

3. AED is indicated for infants as well as pediatric and adult patients in cardiac arrest.

4. Avoid hyperventilation.

    i.   Patients with a pulse but inadequate breathing

        ➤ Adults: 1 breath every 5 to 6 seconds (10 to 12 breaths per minute)

        ➤ Infants and pediatric patients: 1 breath every 3 to 5 seconds (12 to 20 breaths per minute)

    ii. Patients with advanced airway

        ➤ 1 breath every 6 seconds (10 breaths per minute).

        ➤ No pause in compressions with advanced airway

C. Automated External Defibrillation (AEDs)

1. Types of AEDs

    i.   Fully automated external defibrillators. These AEDs do not require the operator to push a button to deliver a shock.

    ii. Semi-automated external defibrillators. These AEDs will not shock until the operator pushes the shock button.

2. Features of AEDs

    i.   Most have two buttons: power and shock.

    ii. Adult and pediatric pads for hands-free defibrillation.

    iii. Visual and audio prompts.

3. Indications: pulseless infant, child, or adult patient

4. Contraindications

   i. Unsafe environment

   ii. Any patient with signs of circulation

5. Utilizing AED

   i. Follow standard assessment guidelines, confirm cardiac arrest, and safe conditions for use of the AED.

   ii. Initiate CPR; obtain an AED.

   iii. Turn on the AED and follow prompts.

   iv. Apply the AED.

      ➤ Expose the chest.

      ➤ Remove medication patches and piercings as needed.

      ➤ Dry the chest if wet; shave excessive hair as needed.

      ➤ Apply appropriate pads per manufacturer's instructions.

         — Sternum/apex position

         — Anterior/posterior position

         — Biaxillary position

      ➤ Avoid placing pads directly over pacemaker, implanted defibrillator, etc.

   v. Deliver shock as indicated. Ensure everyone is clear prior to delivery of shock.

   vi. Resume CPR immediately.

   vii. Re-analyze following two minutes of CPR.

   viii. Initiate transport after third shock or "no-shock" advisory, or per local protocol.

6. Special circumstances

   i. Hypothermic patients should typically be transported after only one shock. Follow local protocol.

   ii. AEDs cannot typically be used in a moving ambulance.

   iii. For witnessed cardiac arrest, the AED should be utilized ASAP. For unwitnessed arrest, it is also acceptable to perform two minutes of CPR before utilizing the AED.

iv. Pediatric AED pads should be used on pediatric patients; however, adult pads should be used if pediatric pads are not available and ALS rescuers are not present with a manual defibrillator.

7. Automated chest compression devices. There are numerous devices on the market, but most are not in widespread use in the United States and are not yet recommended by the American Heart Association in most situations.

D. Withholding Resuscitation

1. Follow local protocol and consult medical direction; however, there are usually only four reasons to withhold resuscitation (the four "Ds"):

   i. Decapitation

   ii. Dependent lividity: blood pooling in the most gravity-dependent area of the body

   iii. Decomposition

   iv. A Do Not Resuscitate (DNR) order

2. For nonsalvageable patients, the focus shifts to providing support for the family.

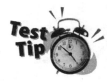

> *Know the current guidelines for CPR. These guidelines will be included on the NREMT exam. If you are unsure about your knowledge of the guidelines, you should review the American Heart Association's Basic Life Support Manual or an equivalent publication. If you are unsure whether your current CPR credential meets the NREMT requirements for certification, contact the NREMT through its website: www.nremt.org.*

PRACTICE QUESTIONS

1. Shock, or hypoperfusion, describes a state of

   A. hypotension.

   B. hypoxia.

   C. inadequate tissue perfusion.

   D. irreversible system collapse.

2. Your trauma patient has lost an unknown amount of blood. The patient is alert, his pulse rate is slightly elevated, and his BP is normal. Based on this information, the patient is most likely experiencing

   A. compensated shock.

   B. anaphylactic shock.

   C. decompensated shock.

   D. neurogenic shock.

3. You are assessing your patient for signs and symptoms of shock. You note tachycardia and pale, cool skin. These findings are

   A. signs of impending circulatory collapse.

   B. indications the patient is not in shock.

   C. examples of the body's defense mechanisms.

   D. not likely related to the patient's state of shock.

4. Your patient presents with signs and symptoms of hypoperfusion. You note the patient's blood pressure is lower each time you reassess vitals. This indicates the patient

   A. is adequately compensating.

   B. is in irreversible shock.

   C. has undiscovered injuries.

   D. is in decompensated shock.

5. Which of the following statements regarding shock in pediatric patients is correct?

   A. Pediatric patients rarely develop shock.

   B. Pediatric patients can be in serious danger and still present without hypotension.

   C. Pediatric patients tend to become hypotensive even during compensated shock.

   D. Signs of shock with hypotension are not usually serious in pediatric patients.

ANSWERS

1. **C.**

   Shock (hypoperfusion) is a state of inadequate tissue perfusion.

2. **A.**

   The patient presents with compensated hemorrhagic shock.

3. **C.**

   The body's compensatory (defense) mechanisms against shock include increased heart rate and peripheral vasoconstriction (leading to pale, cool skin).

4. **D.**

   A falling blood pressure is a sign of decompensated shock. It does not necessarily indicate irreversible shock of undiscovered injuries.

5. **B.**

   Pediatric patients can maintain their blood pressure until about half of their blood volume has been lost. Signs of shock with hypotension in the pediatric population are ominous.

Respiratory Emergencies

Note: Before proceeding with this chapter, review chapters 7 and 9 for the anatomy of the respiratory system.

I. RESPIRATORY DISTRESS

A. Signs and Symptoms of Respiratory Distress: dyspnea, abnormal breathing rate or rhythm, abnormal lung sounds, altered level of consciousness (LOC), accessory muscle use, difficulty speaking, pulse oximeter below 94%, cyanosis, shallow breathing, unequal rise and fall of the chest, thoracic trauma

B. Accessory Muscle Usage: intercostal retractions, abdominal breathing, supraclavicular retractions, tracheal tugging, sternal retractions, nasal flaring, tripod positional breathing, seesaw breathing, pursed-lip breathing

II. CAUSES OF RESPIRATORY EMERGENCIES

A. There are many causes of respiratory emergencies.

1. Causes can be due to medical conditions or traumatic injuries.

2. Some causes are chronic, and others are acute.

3. Any patient complaining of respiratory distress should be evaluated by a higher medical authority. Even patients with subtle signs or symptoms of respiratory problems should be taken seriously.

B. Causes of respiratory complaints include the following:

1. Airway obstruction (Review chapter 9 and your CPR reference text.)

2. Anaphylaxis. Onset can be almost immediate, and is usually within 30 minutes of exposure to an allergen. (Review chapter 13 for additional information.)

3. Asthma

   i. An acute condition caused by bronchoconstriction and excess mucus production. It can be triggered by exercise, allergic response, illness.

   ii. Signs and symptoms include wheezing primarily upon exhalation, absent lung sounds in severe cases, and coughing.

4. Chronic obstructive pulmonary disease (COPD)

   i. A slow, chronic disease process that obstructs and damages the lower airways and alveoli. COPD disorders include chronic bronchitis and emphysema.

      ➤ Several causes, but largely due to cigarette smoking. COPD is chronic, so patients always experience some symptoms of the disease.

   ii. Signs and symptoms

      ➤ History of smoking or exposure to cigarette smoke, chronic productive cough, prolonged expiratory phase, abnormal lung sounds. COPD patients are often on home or portable oxygen.

5. Congestive heart failure (CHF). CHF is a cardiac emergency in which the heart does not pump effectively, leading to a backup of fluid and pulmonary edema. (See chapter 15 for additional information.)

6. Croup

   i. Croup (laryngotracheobronchitis) is inflammation of the pharynx, larynx, and trachea. It is highly infectious and usually occurs in children up to about three years of age.

   ii. Signs and symptoms

      ➤ Croup is usually preceded by a cold and usually occurs in winter.

      ➤ Croup often presents with a unique "barking" cough.

> ➤ Croup often presents with stridor (a high-pitched sound in the upper airway).

7. Cystic fibrosis (CF)

    i.   Genetic disorder leading to thick mucus production and chronic lung infections. Cystic fibrosis often causes death prior to entering adulthood.

    ii. Signs and symptoms include asthma-like symptoms and gastrointestinal problems.

8. Flail chest. See chapter 27.

9. Pneumonia

    i.   Pneumonia is an infection of the lungs. It is often a secondary infection and is a leading cause of pediatric deaths worldwide. Pneumonia is a concern for any patient that aspirates.

    ii. Signs and symptoms

    > ➤ Often history of chronic or terminal illness, productive cough, weakness, chest pain, fever, low pulse oximeter reading.

10. Pneumothorax

    i.   Pneumothorax is the accumulation of air in the pleural space.

    > ➤ It can occur spontaneously, or as a result of trauma.

    > ➤ Asthma patients are at high risk for spontaneous pneumothorax.

    ii. Signs and symptoms

    > ➤ Possible history of respiratory problems or thoracic trauma

    > ➤ Diminished or absent lung sounds in affected area

11. Pulmonary edema

    i.   Pulmonary edema is the accumulation of fluid in the lungs. Causes include CHF, toxic inhalation, disease, and trauma.

    ii. Signs and symptoms include possible cardiac history, rales, pedal edema (swelling in the feet, ankles), and orthopnea (difficulty breathing while lying down).

EMBOLISM

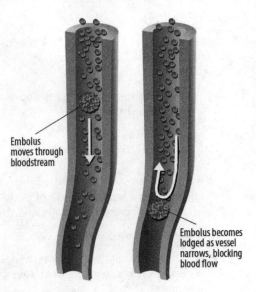

Embolus
moves through
bloodstream

Embolus becomes
lodged as vessel
narrows, blocking
blood flow

Figure 14.1

12. Pulmonary embolism (PE)

   i. PE is the blockage of a pulmonary artery due to a blood clot or other obstruction.

   ii. Signs and symptoms include possible history of recent surgery, or long bone fracture, chest pain, tachypnea, chest pain, hemoptysis, and sudden cardiac arrest.

13. Respiratory syncytial virus (RSV)

   i. RSV is a respiratory infection very common in infants and children. It is extremely contagious. The virus can survive on surfaces, clothing, etc.

   ii. Signs and symptoms include cold-like symptoms, poor fluid intake, and signs of dehydration.

14. Hyperventilation syndrome

   i. Hyperventilation syndrome is characterized by rapid breathing and is often associated with distraught patients.

ii. Hyperventilation syndrome can be a sign of serious underlying medical problems.

iii. Attempt to calm patient, remove from stressful situation.

iv. *Never* have patient breathe into a paper bag or oxygen mask without oxygen.

15. Sucking chest wound. See chapter 27.

16. Thoracic trauma (rib injury, pulmonary contusion, etc.). See chapter 27.

17. Toxic substance exposure. See chapter 19.

III. ASSESSMENT AND MANAGEMENT

(See summary of assessment in chapter 12.)

A. Always take seriously any patient complaining of dyspnea, regardless of the level of distress.

B. Consider continuous positive airway pressure (CPAP), bilevel positive airway pressure (BiPAP), and metered-dose inhaler (MDI) or small-volume nebulizer (SVN) medications per local protocol and with approval of medical direction.

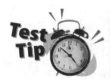

When you are studying the specific medical conditions in these chapters, be sure you understand the pathophysiology of each condition presented.

Suggestion: Write a flashcard for each condition similar to the example below. The answer should be short (two to three sentences maximum) and in terms you understand.

Question: *Describe the pathophysiology of shock.*

Answer: *Shock is inadequate tissue perfusion due to a pump (heart), pipe (vessels), or fluid (blood volume) problem.*

PRACTICE QUESTIONS

1. Which of the following is a slow disease process that obstructs and damages the lower airways and alveoli?

   A. asthma

   B. foreign body airway obstruction

   C. croup

   D. COPD

2. Which of the following is an emergency in which the heart does not pump effectively, leading to a backup of fluid and pulmonary edema?

   A. emphysema

   B. asthma

   C. CHF

   D. COPD

3. Laryngotracheobronchitis is also known as

   A. croup

   B. RSV

   C. CF

   D. emphysema

4. Which of the following are signs and symptoms of a pulmonary embolism?

   A. A history of chronic or terminal illness, productive cough, weakness, low pulse oximeter reading

   B. A history of respiratory problems, thoracic trauma, and absent lung sounds.

   C. A possible history of recent surgery, or long bone fracture, chest pain, tachypnea

   D. A possible cardiac history, rales, pedal edema, and orthopnea

5. Which of the following is characterized by rapid breathing and is often associated with distraught patients?

   A. chronic obstructive pulmonary edema

   B. hyperventilation syndrome

   C. RSV

   D. COPD

ANSWERS

1. **D.**

   COPD is a slow, chronic disease process that obstructs and damages the lower airways and alveoli.

2. **C.**

   Congestive heart failure (CHF) is a cardiac emergency in which the heart does not pump effectively, leading to a backup of fluid and pulmonary edema.

3. **A.**

   Croup (laryngotracheobronchitis) is inflammation of the pharynx, larynx, and trachea.

4. **C.**

   Option A describes pneumonia. Option B describes a pneumothorax. Option D describes a pulmonary embolism.

5. **B.**

   Hyperventilation syndrome is characterized by rapid breathing and is often associated with distraught patients.

Cardiac Emergencies

> *Note:* Before proceeding with this chapter, review chapter 7 for the anatomy of the circulatory system.

I. CARDIAC EMERGENCIES

A. Acute Coronary Syndrome (ACS)

1. Symptoms of ACS are caused by myocardial ischemia (poor blood supply).

2. ACS includes angina pectoris and acute myocardial infarction.

B. Angina Pectoris

1. Angina is transient chest pain caused by a lack of oxygen to the heart muscle. The heart's oxygen demand temporarily exceeds its supply.

   i. Angina is usually caused by atherosclerosis in the coronary arteries.

      ➤ Atherosclerosis is the buildup of plaque in a blood vessel, which can restrict or obstruct blood flow.

   ii. Angina usually occurs during physical activity or stress and resolves with rest, oxygen, or nitroglycerin. Angina does not usually last longer than 10 minutes. Angina does not cause permanent cardiac damage.

2. Signs and symptoms. Presentation is very similar to acute myocardial infarction.

C. Acute Myocardial Infarction (AMI or MI)

1. MI is death to an area of the myocardial muscle due to lack of oxygenated blood flow through the coronary arteries. Dead myocardial muscle cells become scar tissue and cannot contribute to cardiac contraction. Time to restoration of blood flow through coronary arteries is critical to minimizing cardiac damage.

2. Signs and symptoms

   i.   Chest pain or pressure, nausea

   ii.   Weakness, fatigue

   iii. Dyspnea, diaphoresis (excessive sweating)

   iv.   Abnormal vital signs, sudden cardiac arrest

   v.   Patient's denial of the possibility of cardiac emergency or a feeling of impending doom

3. Angina versus MI

   i.   Always treat patient as if chest pain is due to an MI, not angina.

   ii.   MI pain does not usually go away within a few minutes.

   iii. MI pain can occur at any time, not just during exertion.

   iv.   Rest, oxygen, and nitroglycerin may not relieve MI pain.

4. Atypical presentations of MI

   i.   Not all patients experiencing an MI have chest pain.

   ➤ Some patients experience "silent MI" (no pain).

   ➤ Some complain of epigastric pain or indigestion.

   ii.   Patient groups that often experience atypical MI presentations

   ➤ Geriatrics

   ➤ Women

   ➤ Diabetics

   ➤ Alcoholics

5. Complications of MI

   i.   Cardiac dysrhythmias (may cause irregular vitals or sudden cardiac arrest)

   ii.   Sudden cardiac arrest (often before arriving at the hospital)

    iii. Congestive heart failure (due to decreased pump efficiency)

    iv. Cardiogenic shock (due to pump failure)

D. Congestive Heart Failure (CHF)

  1. CHF occurs when the ventricles are unable to keep up with the flow of blood coming to them.

  2. Signs and symptoms

    i. Dyspnea, chest pain, pulmonary edema, JVD, pedal edema

    ii. Orthopnea (difficulty breathing when lying down)

  3. Left versus right ventricular failure

    i. Right ventricular failure

      ➤ If the right ventricle pumps inefficiently, blood backs up into the venous system that feeds into the right heart.

      ➤ Signs include jugular venous distention (JVD), pedal edema.

    ii. Left ventricular failure

      ➤ If the left ventricle pumps inefficiently, blood backs up into the lungs.

      ➤ Signs include pulmonary edema.

        — Pulmonary veins fill due to back pressure.

        — Pressure increases in the pulmonary capillaries.

        — Water leaks from pulmonary capillaries into the alveoli.

      ➤ Left heart failure frequently leads to right heart failure.

E. Hypertension (High Blood Pressure)

  1. A systolic pressure above 140 mmHg or a diastolic pressure above 90 mmHg is considered hypertensive.

  2. Assess for signs or symptoms of a hypertensive crisis.

    i. Hypertensive crises typically involve a blood pressure over 160 systolic or over 94 diastolic.

      ➤ The patient may have associated symptoms or be asymptomatic.

> ➤ Even asymptomatic patients should be evaluated by a physician.

   ii.   Signs and symptoms

> ➤ Headache, often severe

> ➤ Tinnitus: ringing in the ears

> ➤ Nausea and vomiting, dizziness, nosebleed

   3.   Hypertension is a modifiable risk factor with diet, exercise, medications. Left untreated, it can lead to stroke or aortic aneurysm (weakening of aortic wall).

F. Cardiogenic Shock. See chapter 13.

II. ASSESSMENT AND MANAGEMENT
(See summary of assessment in chapter 12.)

A. Any patient with chest pain or other signs and symptoms of a cardiac emergency should be considered a high transport priority.

B. Consider medications such as nitroglycerin and aspirin per local protocol and with approval if medical direction.

C. Consider continuous positive airway pressure (CPAP) or bilevel positive airway pressure (BiPAP) for CHF.

III. AUTOMATIC IMPLANTED CARDIAC DEFIBRILLATORS (AICD) AND PACEMAKERS

A. AICD

   1.   An AICD is similar to an automated external defibrillator (AED), but is placed under the skin and connected directly to the heart.

   2.   Energy output of an AICD is much lower than that of an AED, so it presents minimal risk to providers.

   3.   Treat patients with AICD as you would any other patient. However, if applying an AED, avoid placing pads directly over the device.

B. Pacemaker

1. A pacemaker is an implanted device that helps regulate a patient's cardiac rate and rhythm by serving as an artificial source of electrical impulses to stimulate the heart.

2. Patients with malfunctioning pacemakers often experience dizziness, weakness, bradycardia, or hypotension.

3. Treat patients with a pacemaker as you would any other patient; however, if applying an AED, avoid placing pads directly over device.

IV. RISK FACTORS FOR HEART DISEASE

A. The best approach to cardiac emergencies is prevention through modification of risk factors.

B. Non-modifiable risk factors: Race, Age, Sex, Heredity (**RASH**).

C. Modifiable risk factors: Smoking, Hypertension, Exercise, Diet and diabetes, Stress (**SHEDS**).

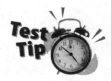

Questions selected for inclusion on the NREMT exam likely fall into one or both of the following categories:

1. The question relates to a task that is performed frequently by the EMT.

2. The question relates to a task that could harm the patient if not performed competently by the EMT.

PRACTICE QUESTIONS

1. Which of the following statements regarding angina is correct?

   A. You should always assume a patient with chest pain is experiencing angina.

   B. Angina pain typically lasts at least 30 minutes.

   C. Angina usually occurs during physical activity or stress.

   D. EMTs can administer naloxone to reduce pain from angina.

2. Your patient is experiencing orthopnea. This means the patient has

   A. difficulty breathing while lying down.

   B. distended neck veins while seated.

   C. increased dyspnea at night

   D. acute swelling of the feet or ankles.

3. Which of the following most likely indicates right ventricular failure?

   A. rales

   B. dyspnea

   C. JVD

   D. orthopnea

4. Your patient has a blood pressure of 146/94. This is considered

   A. hypotensive.

   B. hypertensive.

   C. normotensive.

   D. tachycardia

5. Which of the following is a modifiable risk factor for heart disease?

   A. race

   B. heredity

   C. gender

   D. diabetes

ANSWERS

1. **C.**

   Angina is transient and usually occurs during physical activity or stress and resolves with rest, oxygen, or nitroglycerin (not naloxone). Always treat your patient as if chest pain is due to an MI, not angina.

2. **A.**

   Orthopnea is difficulty breathing while lying down. Distended neck veins is JVD. Increased dyspnea at night is nocturnal dyspnea. Swelling of the feet or ankles is pedal edema.

3. **C.**

   JVD and pedal edema are indications of possible right ventricular failure. Dyspnea and rales are indications of possible left ventricular failure.

4. **B.**

   A systolic pressure above 140 mmHg or a diastolic pressure above 90 mmHg is considered hypertensive.

5. **D.**

   Modifiable risk factors include smoking, hypertension, exercise, diet, diabetes, and stress.

Neurologic Emergencies and Syncope

Chapter 16

I. STROKE

A. Death to brain tissue due to an interruption in blood flow.

1. Also called cerebrovascular accident (CVA) or "brain attack."

2. Modern treatment can dramatically reduce the amount of damage and resulting disability if received in time.

B. Ischemic Strokes

1. Blood flow to the brain is compromised due to a blockage.

2. Ischemic strokes are often due to atherosclerosis.

3. Overwhelming majority of strokes are ischemic in nature.

C. Hemorrhagic Strokes

1. Caused by bleeding within the brain.

2. The bleeding robs the brain of oxygen delivery, and can apply pressure to surrounding brain tissue, further compromising oxygenation.

3. Hemorrhagic strokes limit certain interventions and are often fatal.

4. Prevention through modification of risk factors, especially hypertension, is key.

D. Risk factors for stroke are the same as those for heart disease.

1. Nonmodifiable risk factors: **R**ace, **A**ge, **S**ex, **H**eredity (**RASH**)

2. Modifiable risk factors: **S**moking, **H**ypertension, **E**xercise, **D**iet and diabetes, **S**tress (**SHEDS**)

E. Signs and Symptoms of Stroke

1. Severe headache, slurred speech

2. Facial droop, drooling

3. Unilateral (one-sided) numbness, weakness, or paralysis

4. Altered level of consciousness, difficulty moving or walking

5. Vision problems

F. Stroke Scales

1. Stroke scales are assessments to help identify the probability of a stroke.

2. Performed correctly, they are highly accurate.

3. A locally approved prehospital stroke scale should be performed on any patient suspected of having a stroke.

   i. Cincinnati Prehospital Stroke Scale

   ➤ Facial droop

   — Ask the patient to smile.

   — Abnormal: facial droop is present.

   ➤ Arm drift

   — Ask the patient to close eyes while holding arms out front, palms up.

   — Abnormal: one arm drifts unintentionally.

   ➤ Speech

   — Ask the patient to repeat a given sentence.

   — Abnormal: speech is slurred, word choice is incorrect, or patient is unable to speak.

   ii. Los Angeles Prehospital Stroke Screen: similar to Cincinnati Stroke Scale, but more in-depth.

G. Assessment and Management of the Stroke Patient (See summary of assessment in chapter 12.)

1. Any patient with signs and symptoms of a stroke should be considered a high transport priority and taken to an approved stroke center per local protocol.

2. Protect patient from further harm during movement and transport.

II. TRANSIENT ISCHEMIC ATTACK (TIA)

A. TIAs have the same presentation as a CVA. However, the signs and symptoms self-correct within about 24 hours with no permanent brain damage.

B. TIAs are also called mini strokes.

C. TIAs are a warning sign of an impending stroke.

III. SEIZURES

A. Seizures are caused by disorganized electrical activity within the brain.

B. Types of Seizures

   1. Generalized seizures

     i. Also called grand mal seizures.

     ii. Patient is unresponsive and experiences full-body convulsions.

   2. Absence seizures

     i. Also called petit mal seizures.

     ii. Patient does not interact with environment, but there is no convulsive activity.

   3. Partial seizures

     i. Simple partial seizure: no change in level of consciousness (LOC); possible twitching or sensory changes, but no full-body convulsions

     ii. Complex partial seizures: altered LOC; isolated twitching and sensory changes possible

   4. Status epilepticus

     i. Prolonged seizure (about 30 minutes) or recurring seizures without the patient regaining consciousness in between

     ii. Highly dangerous, possibly leading to permanent brain damage and death

C. Phases of a Seizure

1. Not every stage is present for every type of seizure or every patient.

2. Aura phase

    i.   This is the warning stage.

    ii. The patient may sense onset of seizure.

3. Tonic phase

    i.   Muscle rigidity

    ii. Possible incontinence

4. Tonic-clonic phase

    i.   Patient experiences uncontrolled muscle contraction and relaxation.

    ii. Patient may be apneic during the tonic or tonic-clonic phase.

5. Postictal phase

    i.   This is the "recovery" phase.

    ii. Patient's LOC progressively improves over about 30 minutes.

D. Causes of Seizures

1. Seizures can be caused by congenital problems, traumatic injuries, or medical conditions, including alcohol, brain injury, tumor, diabetic emergency, epilepsy, fever, infection, insulin or other medications, poisoning or toxic exposure, stroke, or biological or chemical weapons.

2. Febrile seizures are a common cause of seizures in pediatric patients. Caused by high fevers that develop rapidly, they do not typically present significant risk to the patient. The child should, however, be transported and evaluated by a physician.

3. Recognizing seizures

    i.   Often, EMS providers will not arrive until the patient is in the postictal phase.

    ii. Question bystanders.

    iii. Assess for incontinence, tongue biting.

    iv. Obtain thorough history, medications, etc., when able.

4. Management of seizure patients. (See summary of assessment in chapter 12.)

   If possible, position postictal patient in the lateral recumbent position to protect airway. If vomiting occurs while in cervical-spine precautions, tilt the long board.

IV. SYNCOPE

A. Syncope is fainting.

B. It is typically caused by a temporary loss of blood flow to the brain.

C. Causes include cardiac emergency, hypotension, neurological problem, stress, diabetes, pregnancy, anemia, medications, and toxic exposure.

D. Patients typically regain consciousness as soon as they are supine and blood flow returns to the brain.

E. Assessment and Management (See summary of assessment in chapter 12.)

   1. When in doubt, err on the side of caution and encourage treatment and transport for a patient experiencing a syncopal episode.

   2. Consider assistance from ALS providers or contact medical direction.

V. HEADACHE

A. Headaches have many causes, some of them neurological.

B. A few causes of headache include stroke, aneurysm, tumor, hypertension, migraines, trauma, and meningitis.

C. Signs and symptoms of possible medical emergency include severe headache, hypertension, fever, stiff neck, neurological impairment, or recent trauma.

D. Assessment and Management (See summary of assessment in chapter 12.)

    1. When in doubt, err on the side of caution and encourage treatment and transport for a patient with a headache.

    2. Consider assistance from ALS providers or contact medical direction.

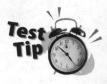

> *The higher a task's potential for harm, the more likely it is to appear on the certification exam. You will likely see many questions related to interventions that have a high risk of harm to the patient if performed inappropriately. These questions are preferred by the NREMT over questions related to tasks that pose little risk of harm.*
>
> *Be sure your preparation for the certification exam includes a review of interventions with the potential to cause harm. Simply put, if it is important to know when taking care of your patients, then it is important to know before taking the certification exam.*

PRACTICE QUESTIONS

1. Death of brain tissue due to an interruption in blood flow is known as

    A. a transient ischemic attack.

    B. a stroke.

    C. a myocardial infarction.

    D. acute coronary syndrome.

2. Which of the following is part of the Cincinnati Prehospital Stroke Scale?

    A. blood pressure

    B. distal pulses

    C. arm drift

    D. blood glucose

3. Your patient is unresponsive and experiencing full-body convulsions. The patient is presenting with

   A. absence seizures

   B. generalized seizures

   C. petit mal seizures

   D. partial seizures

4. Which of the following presents the greatest danger to the patient?

   A. status epilepticus

   B. complex partial seizure

   C. petit mal seizure

   D. simple partial seizure

5. Which of the following patients is most likely to experience a febrile seizure?

   A. A 65-year-old patient

   B. A 17-year-old patient

   C. A 35-year-old patient

   D. A 4-month-old patient

ANSWERS

1. **B.**

   Death of brain tissue due to an interruption in blood flow is known as a stroke, cerebrovascular accident (CVA), or "brain attack."

2. **C.**

   The Cincinnati Prehospital Stroke Scale assesses facial droop, arm drift, and speech.

3. **B.**

   Generalized (grand mal) seizures are characterized by unresponsiveness and full-body convulsions.

4. A.

Status epilepticus seizures are highly dangerous, possibly leading to permanent brain damage and death.

5. D.

Febrile seizures are a common cause of seizures in pediatric patients.

Diabetic Emergencies

I. METABOLISM AND ENERGY PRODUCTION

A. Energy Sources

   1. Sugars (glucose)

   2. Fat

   3. Protein

B. Glucose

   1. Glucose it the body's primary fuel source.

   2. It is the only fuel source used by the brain.

   3. In addition to oxygen, the brain must have a continuous supply of glucose.

   4. Use of glucose as a fuel source is an aerobic (with oxygen) function. The body is well equipped to deal with by-products of aerobic metabolism (water, carbon dioxide).

C. Fats and Proteins

   1. The brain cannot use these alternate fuel sources, but the rest of the body can.

   2. These energy sources are used in an anaerobic (without oxygen) environment.

   3. Fats and proteins are far less efficient (by about 19 times) than glucose fuel source.

   4. By-products of anaerobic metabolism (ketones) are dangerous.

II. INSULIN, GLUCAGON, AND BLOOD GLUCOSE LEVELS

A. Insulin and Blood Glucose

1. Sugars enter the body and quickly reach the bloodstream. Blood glucose levels can be checked using a glucometer.

2. Insulin (a pancreatic hormone) is needed to efficiently move glucose out of the bloodstream and into the cells to provide energy.

3. Insulin will cause blood glucose levels to drop as glucose leaves the bloodstream and enters the cells.

4. Without insulin, glucose cannot enter the cells efficiently and blood glucose levels will rise. The cells begin to starve and look for other fuel sources.

5. While most cells in the body begin looking for alternate fuel sources, brain cells cannot.

6. While the brain can use only glucose as an energy source, it has the ability to accept glucose with or without insulin. As a result

    i. brain cells will starve and begin to die if there is no glucose, regardless of the presence of alternate fuel sources, such as fat and protein

    ii. brain cells will *not* starve if there is glucose present, regardless of the presence of insulin

B. Glucagon and Blood Glucose Levels

1. Glucagon (also a pancreatic hormone) works opposite of insulin.

2. Glucagon serves to increase blood glucose levels.

III. NORMAL GLUCOSE REGULATION

The normal process for regulation of blood glucose is cyclical.

A. Food is consumed and the blood glucose rises.

B. Insulin is released and glucose is transported into cells.

C. Blood glucose levels fall and glucagon is released.

D. Glucagon acts to temporarily maintain blood glucose levels.

E. Food is consumed and the process continues.

IV. TESTING BLOOD GLUCOSE

A. A glucometer is used to assess capillary blood glucose levels.

B. In the United States, glucometers measure blood glucose levels in milligrams per deciliter (mg/dL).

C. Normal level is 80 to 120 mg/dL. However, 120 to 140 mg/dL is not unusual after eating.

D. Hypoglycemia is a blood glucose of 60 mg/dL or less.

E. Hyperglycemia is a sustained blood glucose greater than about 120 mg/dL.

V. PATHOPHYSIOLOGY OF DIABETES MELLITUS

A. Diabetes is a disease caused by an inability to metabolize glucose normally. This is frequently due to a problem with insulin production. Untreated diabetics typically have elevated blood glucose levels due to a lack of insulin or ineffective insulin.

 1. As blood glucose levels approach about 200 mg/dL, glucose begins to spill into the urine.

 2. Glucose draws water, so increased urinary output and dehydration is common. Dehydration leads to thirst, and cells starving for glucose stimulate hunger.

B. Type I Diabetes

 1. Also called insulin-dependent diabetes mellitus (IDDM).

 2. Type I diabetics must take (usually inject) supplemental insulin.

3. Type I diabetes usually develops in pediatric patients.

4. Type I diabetes appears to be genetically caused in most cases.

5. Untreated type I diabetics will present with the three "P's" (explained below) and very high blood glucose levels.

6. Type I diabetics are at high risk for diabetic ketoacidosis (DKA) if untreated.

7. Type I diabetics are at high risk for insulin shock due to insulin overdose.

C. Type II Diabetes

1. Also knows as non-insulin-dependent diabetes mellitus (NIDDM).

2. Type II diabetics do not typically require supplemental insulin.

3. Type II diabetes is caused by a combination of lifestyle and genetics. It can be largely controlled through diet, exercise, and oral medications.

4. Type II is more common than type I diabetes.

5. Incidence of type II diabetes is growing rapidly in the United States, largely due to obesity.

D. The three "P's" are the triad of classic symptoms for untreated diabetic emergencies related to hyperglycemia.

1. Polyuria: excessive urination due to excess glucose in the urine

2. Polydipsia: excessive thirst due to dehydration

3. Polyphagia: excessive hunger due to cell starvation

E. Risks of Diabetes

1. Fatty deposits in blood vessels increase risk of stroke and heart attack.

2. Chronically high blood glucose levels can damage arteries, compromising circulation and leading to blindness and amputation of lower extremities.

3. Poor circulation can lead to ulcers and difficulty healing.

VI. SPECIFIC DIABETIC EMERGENCIES

A. Hypoglycemia and Insulin Shock

   1. Hypoglycemia

      i. A blood glucose level below 60 mg/dL with signs and symptoms or a blood glucose level below 50 mg/dL regardless of the presence of signs or symptoms.

      ii. Occurs more often in type I diabetes than type II diabetes.

      iii. Hypoglycemia can very quickly lead to an altered level of consciousness (LOC), seizures, coma, and brain death.

   2. Insulin shock

      i. "Insulin shock" is a term commonly used to refer to severe hypoglycemia with signs and symptoms.

      ii. Diabetics can suddenly become confused, violent, or unresponsive due to severe hypoglycemia.

      iii. Commonly caused by a sudden unexpected drop in blood glucose due to

        ➤ taking a regular insulin dose but not eating

        ➤ extreme physical activity without adjusting insulin level or food intake

        ➤ insulin overdose

   3. Signs and symptoms of hypoglycemia/insulin shock

      i. Onset of signs and symptoms is typically rapid. Brain damage can occur rapidly. Treatment must be provided rapidly.

      ii. Low blood glucose level.

      iii. Signs and symptoms caused by brain cell starvation

        ➤ Altered LOC, such as confusion or irritability

        ➤ Seizures or coma

      iv. Signs and symptoms caused by an increase in epinephrine release (this shuts down release of insulin and stimulates release of glucagon)

        ➤ Possible restlessness, anxiousness, irritability

> ➤ Diaphoresis, tachycardia

> ➤ Pale, cool skin, tremors

v. Patients with hypoglycemia are often misdiagnosed as being intoxicated or a behavioral emergency.

B. Hyperglycemia and Diabetic Ketoacidosis

1. Hyperglycemia

    i. A sustained blood glucose over 120 mg/dL.

    ii. Hyperglycemia typically develops slowly and requires a slower recovery process.

    iii. Hyperglycemic patients can experience seizures, coma, and permanent injury; however, they do not typically develop signs and symptoms rapidly as do hypoglycemic patients.

2. Diabetic ketoacidosis (DKA)

    i. Occurs more frequently with type I diabetes.

    ii. With DKA, the blood glucose is frequently above 350 mg/dL.

    iii. Brain cells are able to utilize glucose, but the rest of the body's cells are starving and begin using alternate fuel sources.

    iv. The body spills large amounts of glucose into the urine, which increases urinary output and leads to dehydration.

    v. The use of alternate fuel sources (anaerobic metabolism) leads to the production of ketones and acidosis.

    vi. It is the acidosis that threatens the brain during DKA, not a lack of glucose.

3. Signs and symptoms of DKA

    i. High blood glucose, typically above 350 mg/dL

    ii. Kussmaul respirations: deep, rapid breaths

    iii. The three "P's"

    > ➤ Polydipsia: excessive thirst

    > ➤ Polyphagia: excessive hunger

    > ➤ Polyuria: excessive urination

iv. Unusual odor on breath: fruity or acetone-like

v. Incontinence

vi. Tachycardia

vii. Coma

4. Hyperglycemic hyperosmolar nonketotic syndrome

i. Similar to DKA, without the buildup of ketones

ii. Occurs more frequently with type II diabetes

VII. MANAGEMENT OF DIABETIC EMERGENCY
(See summary of assessment in chapter 12.)

A. Consider oral glucose if the patient is hypoglycemic and able to swallow.

B. Consult medical direction and follow local protocols for blood glucose testing and administration of oral glucose.

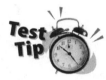

Eighty-five percent of the questions from the first four categories on the NREMT certification exam relate to adult patients; 15% of the questions relate to pediatric patients (see table below). Make sure you are prepared for this!

NREMT Exam Topics	Adult vs. Pediatric Patients
Airway and ventilation	*85% adult*
	15% pediatric
Cardiology, resuscitation, stroke	*85% adult*
	15% pediatric
Trauma	*85% adult*
	15% pediatric
Medical and OB, GYN	*85% adult*
	15% pediatric

Source: NREMT (2017). Test Plan. https://www.nremt.org/rwd/public/document/cognitive-exam

PRACTICE QUESTIONS

1. Insulin will cause blood glucose levels to
   A. fluctuate.
   B. stabilize.
   C. elevate.
   D. drop.

2. Which of the following represents a normal blood glucose level?
   A. 40–60 mg/dL
   B. 80–120 mg/dL
   C. 120–160 mg/dL
   D. 160–200 mg/dL

3. If a patient's blood glucose level exceeds 200 mg/dL, which of the following is most likely?
   A. increased urinary output
   B. acute hypertension
   C. sudden loss of consciousness
   D. decreased respirations

4. Your patient has been experiencing excessive hunger, thirst, and urinary output. You should suspect
   A. insulin shock.
   B. severe hyperglycemia.
   C. moderate hypoglycemia.
   D. an insulin overdose.

5. Your patient has a blood glucose of 370 mg/dL. You should suspect

   A. DKA.

   B. insulin shock.

   C. Type II diabetes.

   D. Type III diabetes.

ANSWERS

1. **D.**

   Insulin will cause blood glucose levels to drop as glucose leaves the bloodstream and enters the cells.

2. **B.**

   A normal blood glucose level is 80 to 120 mg/dL.

3. **A.**

   As blood glucose levels approach about 200 mg/dL, glucose begins to spill into the urine. Glucose draws water, so increased urinary output and dehydration is common.

4. **B.**

   Excessive hunger, thirst, and urination are the triad of classic symptoms for untreated diabetic emergencies related to hyperglycemia.

5. **A.**

   Diabetic ketoacidosis (DKA) occurs more frequently with type I diabetes and the blood glucose is frequently above 350 mg/dL.

Anaphylaxis

I. PATHOPHYSIOLOGY OF ANAPHYLAXIS

A. Immune Response

1. Foreign bodies (antigens) can be absorbed, ingested, injected, or inhaled.

2. Immune system detects antigens and deploys antibodies to fight them.

B. Allergic Reaction

1. Some antigens (allergens) stimulate an allergic reaction.

2. An allergic reaction is an excessive immune response to an allergen.

   i. Allergic reactions can be local or systemic.

   ii. Symptoms include itching, watery eyes, runny nose, etc.

3. Sensitization. Patients can develop sensitivity to a substance that did not previously cause a reaction, such as latex. Following sensitization, the severity of reactions can get progressively worse each time.

C. Anaphylaxis (also known as anaphylactic reaction or anaphylactic shock)

1. Anaphylaxis is a severe, life-threatening form of allergic reaction.

2. Anaphylaxis is always systemic and impairs the airway, respiratory, and cardiovascular systems. Anaphylaxis causes upper- and lower-airway swelling, bronchoconstriction, vasodilation, hypotension, capillary permeability (leakage), and increased mucus production.

II. CAUSES OF ANAPHYLAXIS

A. Medications, such as antibiotics, aspirin, nonsteroidal anti-inflammatory (NSAID) medications, vitamins

B. Environmental triggers, such as chemicals and pollens

C. Foods, including peanut products and derivatives, shellfish, eggs

D. Bites and stings from wasps, bees, ants, etc.

E. Latex (found in many medical supplies)

III. SIGNS AND SYMPTOMS

A. Central nervous system: restlessness, anxious, irritable

B. Skin: flushed, hives, swelling

C. Respiratory: dyspnea, tachypnea, wheezing, stridor

D. Cardiovascular: tachycardia, hypotension

IV. MANAGEMENT
(See summary of patient assessment in chapter 12.)

A. Consider intramuscular (IM) administration of the epinephrine auto-injector per medical direction and local protocol.

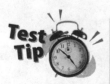

It is essential to understand the impact of vasodilation on anaphylaxis. During anaphylaxis, systemic vasodilation (enlargement of blood vessels) leads to hypotension and distributive shock. It also contributes to capillary permeability (leakage) and pulmonary edema.

Remember:

>   *Vasodilation = enlargement of blood vessels*

>   *Anaphylaxis = massive vasodilation!*

>   *Massive vasodilation = distributive shock!*

PRACTICE QUESTIONS

1. Which of the following statements regarding anaphylaxis is correct?

    A. Anaphylaxis can be a local or systemic medical emergency.

    B. Anaphylaxis impairs primarily endocrine function.

    C. Anaphylaxis is always a systemic emergency.

    D. Anaphylaxis typically causes itchy eyes and runny nose.

2. Anaphylaxis typically causes

    A. hypotension.

    B. hypertension.

    C. bradycardia.

    D. bradypnea.

3. Administration of an epinephrine auto-injector is indicated for

    A. any patient experiencing an allergic reaction.

    B. a patient with obvious local symptoms of an allergic reaction.

    C. patients with signs and symptoms of anaphylaxis.

    D. patients with signs and symptoms of a narcotic overdose.

4. Which of the following is true regarding the epinephrine auto-injector?

    A. The epinephrine auto-injector is administered intravenously.

    B. The epinephrine auto-injector is administered intramuscularly.

    C. The epinephrine auto-injector is administered subcutaneously.

    D. The epinephrine auto-injector is administered transdermally.

5. Patients can develop sensitivity to a substance that did not previously cause a reaction. This is known as

    A. desensitization.

    B. antigen deployment.

    C. an antigen reaction.

    D. sensitization.

ANSWERS

1. **C.**

   Anaphylaxis is always a systemic medical emergency that affects the respiratory and cardiovascular systems. Itchy eyes and runny nose are localized symptoms of an allergic reaction.

2. **A.**

   Anaphylaxis typically causes hypotension, tachycardia, and tachypnea.

3. **C.**

   An epinephrine auto-injector is indicated for patients experiencing anaphylaxis.

4. **B.**

   The epinephrine auto-injector is administered intramuscularly.

5. **D.**

   Sensitization occurs when patients develop sensitivity to a substance that did not previously cause a reaction. Following sensitization, the severity of reactions can get progressively worse.

Toxicology

I. INTRODUCTION

A. Poisonings occur in both adult and pediatric populations.

1. Accidental pediatric poisonings are more common, but less often fatal.

2. Adult poisonings can be accidental or intentional. They are less frequent, but more often fatal.

B. Intentional Abuse of Drugs and Toxins

1. Addiction: a physical or psychological need to continue misusing a drug or toxin

2. Tolerance: the need to take increasing amounts of the drug or toxin to achieve the desired effects

C. Routes of exposure: ingestion, inhalation, injection, and absorption

II. INGESTED TOXINS

A. Ingestion is the most common route of exposure.

B. Examples of ingested poisons include drugs, plants, and household chemicals.

C. Ingestion of poisons by children is usually accidental, but most incidences involving adults are intentional.

D. Prescription and Over-the-Counter Medications

1. Accidental overdose is common, especially in pediatric and geriatric patients.

2. Common accidental overdose medications include cardiac medications, psychiatric medications, and acetaminophen.

3. Prescription narcotics are commonly abused.

E. Other Commonly Ingested Toxins

1. Food. The incidence of food poisonings in the United States has been increasing.

2. Plants. Many plants are poisonous. Examples include oleander, foxglove, castor beans, jasmine, elderberry, mistletoe, nightshade, jimson weed, among many others.

F. Signs and Symptoms. These vary based on what is ingested, but may include

   i.   burning to the mouth and airway with acids or alkalis

   ii. stomach pain, cramps, nausea, vomiting

   iii. altered level of consciousness (LOC)

   iv. altered vital signs, seizures

G. Intentional overdoses by adults often involve more than one substance. Always attempt to determine what else the patient might have taken.

H. Sedatives, Narcotics, Barbiturates

1. Sedatives, narcotics, and barbiturates are commonly abused drugs.

2. All three can cause a decreased LOC and respiratory depression.

3. Many narcotics also cause pupillary constriction.

I. SPECIFIC INTERVENTIONS FOR INGESTED TOXINS

1. Consider activated charcoal per medical direction. (See chapter 11 for additional information about activated charcoal.)

2. Consider contacting medical direction or a Poison Control Center (1-800-222-1222, U.S.) for information about medications you are not familiar with.

III. INHALATION

A. Examples of inhaled poisons include various chemicals, pesticides, carbon monoxide, and natural gas.

B. Signs and Symptoms

   1. The onset of symptoms may be rapid or delayed.

   2. Signs and symptoms may include dyspnea, coughing, dizziness, headache, and abnormal lung sounds.

C. Specific Interventions for Inhaled Toxins

   1. Make sure the scene is safe. Be alert for multiple victims.

   2. Administer high-flow oxygen, and monitor lung sounds and respiratory status carefully.

IV. INJECTION

A. It is difficult to diminish, dilute, or inhibit the effects of injected toxins.

B. Most injected poisonings are due to drug abuse.

C. Onset of effects from injected drugs is typically rapid and can be long-lasting.

D. Be alert for needles.

E. Commonly injected toxins include narcotics (e.g., morphine, heroin) and stimulants (e.g., cocaine, amphetamines).

   1. Signs and symptoms of injected stimulants include the following:

      i. Mood elevation, euphoria

      ii. Restlessness, excitability

      iii. Tachycardia, rebound depression

      iv. Can lead to seizures, heart attack, stroke, death

2. Signs and symptoms of injected narcotics include the following:

    i.   Decreased level of consciousness, respiratory depression

    ii. Possible pupillary constrictio, also known as "pinpoint" pupils

    iii. Can lead to respiratory arrest, seizures, coma, and death

V. ABSORPTION

A. Examples of absorbed poisons include pesticides, various acids and alkalis, and petroleum-based products.

B. Signs and symptoms include burns to the skin, rash or blisters, itching or burning.

C. Specific Interventions for Absorbed Toxins

1. Decontaminate patient appropriately before initiating care or transport.

2. Most chemicals on the skin or in the eyes should be irrigated with water continuously for about 20 minutes.

3. When irrigating the eyes, be sure not to irrigate toxin into unaffected eye.

4. Some (not many) chemicals react with water. Consult *Emergency Response Guidebook*, fire department personnel, hazardous materials team, or medical direction if unsure.

VI. ASSESSMENT AND MANAGEMENT

(See summary of assessment in chapter 12.)

A. Avoid exposure to toxin; remove patient from the source of the toxin if applicable and safe to do so.

B. Decontaminate patient if needed and safe to do so, or request additional resources.

C. Always administer oxygen and check a blood glucose level for any patient with an altered or decreased LOC.

D. Consider naloxone for a suspected narcotic overdose per local protocol and with medical direction approval.

E. Consider activated charcoal for recently ingested poisons per local protocol and with medical direction approval.

 VII. SPECIFIC DRUGS AND TOXINS OF ABUSE

A. Alcohol

   1. Alcohol is the most widely abused drug in the United States.

   2. Most long-term alcoholics will develop hepatitis.

   3. Alcohol is a central nervous system (CNS) depressant and a sedative (calms, tranquilizes) hypnotic (sleep inducing).

   4. Ingestion of alcohol increases risk of vomiting.

   5. Alcohol withdrawal may cause delirium tremens (DTs).

      i.   Restless, irritable, agitated

      ii. Hallucinations, tremors, or seizures

B. Narcotics

   1. Narcotics are widely abused. They are typically ingested or injected.

   2. Narcotics, or opioids, include morphine, codeine, heroin, oxycodone, and many more.

   3. Narcotics are CNS depressants that can cause coma and severe respiratory depression.

C. Sedative Hypnotic Drugs

   1. Sedative hypnotics are CNS depressants.

   2. Sedatives have a calming effect, and hypnotics induce sleep.

   3. Sedative hypnotics are usually taken orally but can be injected.

   4. Barbiturates such as Amytal, Seconal, and Luminal are sedative hypnotics.

   5. Benzodiazepines such as Valium, Xanax, and Rohypnol are sedative hypnotics.

D. Inhalants

1. Abused inhalants may include acetones, glues, cleaning chemicals, paints, hydrocarbons, aerosols, and propellants.

2. These chemicals are inhaled to achieve sedative hypnotic effects.

3. The difference between an effective dose and a lethal dose is very narrow.

4. Brain damage and/or cardiac arrest due to abuse is common.

5. Prescription and over-the-counter bronchodilators are also abused. They are taken for stimulant effects or perceived advantage in competitive sports.

E. Stimulants

1. Stimulants include caffeine, cocaine, amphetamines, methamphetamines, among others.

2. They are taken for stimulant and euphoric effects.

3. They can be taken by any route and are commonly injected, ingested, and inhaled.

F. Marijuana

1. Marijuana (cannabis) is typically smoked.

2. It is taken to induce euphoria, relaxation, drowsiness.

3. Marijuana use does not usually create an acute medical emergency; however, marijuana users often take other illicit drugs.

G. Hallucinogens

1. Hallucinogens alter sensory perception.

2. Examples include LSD and PCP.

H. Carbon monoxide (CO)

1. CO poisoning is a leading cause of death due to fires. Other common sources include home heating devices and vehicle exhaust fumes.

2. Carbon monoxide inhibits the body's ability to transport and use oxygen.

3. The danger of CO poisoning is greatest when exposed in a confined space.

4. Carbon monoxide is a silent killer. It is tasteless, colorless, odorless, and completely nonirritating when inhaled. Victims are usually unaware they are being exposed and eventually lose consciousness.

I. Acids, Alkalis, and Hydrocarbons

   1. Acids and alkalis

      i. Both are considered caustic substances.

      ii. Many household products are acids or alkalis.

      iii. Acids have a very low pH and burn on contact. Pain is usually immediate.

      iv. Alkalis have a very high pH and tend to burn deeper than acids. Pain may be delayed.

      v. Most caustic ingestion patients are children.

      vi. Common household caustics include liquid drain openers, bathroom cleaning supplies, ammonia, and bleach.

   2. Hydrocarbons

      i. Hydrocarbons are petroleum-based.

      ii. Hydrocarbons are found in gasoline, paints, solvents, sunscreen, baby oil, makeup remover, kerosene, lighter fluid, and more.

      iii. Hydrocarbons can be ingested, inhaled, and absorbed.

      iv. Most hydrocarbon ingestion patients are children.

   3. Note that activated charcoal is contraindicated with caustic or hydrocarbon ingestion.

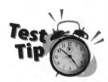

Test Tip

Because the exam is computer-adaptive, you cannot go back and change your answer on a previous question once it is submitted. Make sure you have marked your answer correctly before moving on.

PRACTICE QUESTIONS

1. Which of the following is a physical or psychological need to continue misusing a drug or toxin?

   A. habituation

   B. tolerance

   C. addiction

   D. withdrawal

2. What is the most common route of exposure?

   A. ingestion

   B. inhalation

   C. absorption

   D. injection

3. An overdose on sedatives, barbiturates, or narcotics is most likely to cause

   A. excitation.

   B. tachycardia.

   C. respiratory depression.

   D. hypertension.

4. Your overdose patient has a decreased LOC and "pinpoint" pupils. Which of the following is most likely?

   A. amphetamine overdose

   B. narcotic overdose

   C. cocaine overdose

   D. barbiturate overdose

5. LSD and PCP are

   A. barbiturates.

   B. cannabis.

   C. narcotics.

   D. hallucinogens.

ANSWERS

1. **C.**

   Addiction is a physical or psychological need to continue misusing a drug or toxin. Tolerance is the need to take increasing amounts of the drug or toxin to achieve the desired effects.

2. **A.**

   Ingestion is the most common route of exposure.

3. **C.**

   Sedative, narcotic, and barbiturate overdoses are likely to cause decreased LOC and respiratory depression.

4. **B.**

   Decreased LOC, respiratory depression, and pupillary constriction are common signs of a narcotic overdose. Amphetamines and cocaine are stimulants. Pupillary constriction is not common with barbiturate overdoses.

5. **D.**

   LSD and PCP are hallucinogens.

Abdominal, Gynecologic, and Genitourinary/ Renal Emergencies

I. INTRODUCTION TO ACUTE ABDOMINAL PAIN

A. Acute (sudden onset) abdominal pain is usually due to trauma, distention, inflammation, or ischemia.

B. Types of Abdominal Pain

1. Note that the level of pain does not necessarily indicate the illness's severity. Patients can have a life-threatening abdominal emergency without severe pain.

2. Visceral pain

   i. Dull, diffuse pain that is difficult to localize

   ii. Frequently associated with nausea and vomiting

   iii. Often not severe, but may indicate actual organ injury

3. Parietal pain

   i. Severe, localized pain. Usually sharp and constant.

   ii. The pain will often cause the patient to curl up with knees to chest.

   iii. The patient is often very still and breathing shallowly to diminish pain.

4. Referred pain: causes pain in an area of the body other than the source

II. CAUSES OF ACUTE ABDOMINAL PAIN

A. Appendicitis

1. Caused by inflammation of the appendix.

2. Can lead to life-threatening infection and septic shock.

3. Signs and symptoms

   i. Nausea, vomiting, diarrhea, loss of appetite, fever.

   ii. Pain may begin as diffuse, but usually localizes to right lower quadrant.

B. Peritonitis

1. Peritonitis is caused by inflammation of the peritoneum (membrane lining the abdominal organs and cavity).

2. Signs and symptoms: nausea, vomiting, loss of appetite, diarrhea, fever.

C. Cholecystitis

1. Cholecystitis is inflammation of the gall bladder, often due to gallstones.

2. Most often occurs in females 30 to 50 years of age.

3. Signs and symptoms

   i. Right upper quadrant pain

   ii. Increased pain at night

   iii. Increased pain after eating fatty foods

   iv. Referred pain to the shoulder is common

   v. Nausea and vomiting

D. Diverticulitis

1. Diverticulitis develops when small pouches (diverticula) along the wall of the intestine fill with feces and become inflamed and infected.

2. Typically affects people over age 40 and is associated with a low-fiber diet.

3. Signs and symptoms

   i. Usually abdominal pain in the lower left quadrant

   ii. Fever

      iii. Weakness

      iv. Nausea and vomiting

      v. Bleeding *not* common

E. Gastrointestinal (GI) Bleeding

  1. Most often occurs in middle-aged patients

  2. Most often fatal in geriatric patients

  3. Upper GI bleeds: often due to ulcers

  4. Lower GI bleeds: often due to diverticulitis

  5. Signs and symptoms

      i. Hematemesis: vomiting blood

      ii. Hematochezia: bloody stool

      iii. Dark, tarry stool

      iv. Signs and symptoms of hypovolemic shock

F. Gastroenteritis

  1. Gastroenteritis is an infection with associated diarrhea, nausea, and vomiting.

  2. It is usually due to contaminated food or water and is not contagious.

  3. Prolonged vomiting and diarrhea can lead to hypovolemic shock.

  4. Gastroenteritis is a common cause of shock in children.

G. Esophageal Varices

  1. Esophageal varices are a weakening of the blood vessels lining the esophagus.

  2. The condition is frequently associated with alcoholism.

  3. Signs and symptoms

      i. Vomiting large amounts of bright red blood

      ii. History of alcohol abuse or liver disease

      iii. Signs and symptoms of hypovolemic shock

H. Ulcers

    1. Ulcers are open wounds along the digestive tract, often the stomach.

    2. Signs and symptoms

        i. History of ulcers

        ii. Abdominal pain in the left upper quadrant

        iii. Nausea and vomiting

        iv. Often elicits an increase in pain before meals and during stress

I. ABDOMINAL AORTIC ANEURYSM (AAA)

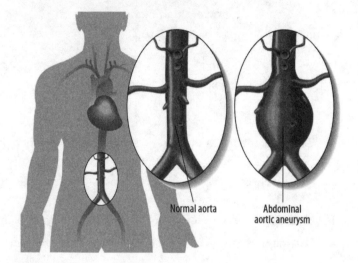

Normal aorta   Abdominal aortic aneurysm

    1. AAA is a weakening of the wall of the aorta in the abdominal region.

    2. Weakened area is prone to rupture. A ruptured AAA will likely cause rapid, fatal bleeding.

    3. Signs and symptoms

        i. AAA most common in geriatric males

        ii. Tearing back pain

        iii. Signs and symptoms of hypovolemic shock

        iv. Possible pulsating abdominal mass

4. Patients with a suspected AAA should be transported to an appropriate facility without delay.

III. GYNECOLOGICAL EMERGENCIES

A. Gynecologic emergencies relate to female patients and their reproductive systems.

B. Abdominal pain is the most common symptom of most gynecologic emergencies.

C. Specific Gynecologic Emergencies

1. Sexual assault

   i. Sexual assault patients have been victimized physically and psychologically.

   ii. Management of sexual assault victims

   ➤ Request law enforcement and victim's assistance.

   ➤ Do not touch the patient without consent.

   ➤ Request a same-sex provider if one is not already on scene.

   ➤ Encourage the patient not to change clothes, shower, etc.

   ➤ Treat clothing as evidence. Do not touch unless necessary.

   ➤ Touch only those things that are necessary.

2. Pelvic inflammatory disease (PID)

   i. PID is painful and requires treatment. Non-emergency transport is recommended.

   ii. Signs and symptoms

   ➤ Abdominal pain

   ➤ Fever

   ➤ Pain during urination

   ➤ Often, increased pain while walking

3. Vaginal bleeding. This condition has many potential causes, including spontaneous abortion, PID, and sexually transmitted diseases.

4. Signs and symptoms of gynecologic problems

    i.   Abdominal pain

    ii. Vaginal bleeding or discharge

    iii. Signs and symptoms of shock

    iv. Fever, nausea, and vomiting

IV. GENITOURINARY AND RENAL EMERGENCIES

A. Urinary Tract Infection (UTI)

1. Signs and symptoms

    i.   Abdominal pain

    ii. Hematuria: blood in urine

    iii. Painful or frequent urination

    iv. Fever, nausea, and vomiting

B. Kidney Stones

1. Kidney stones are crystals formed in the kidneys that can cause an obstruction in the urinary tract, causing severe pain.

2. Males are much more likely to develop kidney stones.

3. Signs and symptoms

    i.   Severe abdominal pain, groin pain

    ii. Painful urination, fever, nausea, and vomiting

C. Kidney Failure

1. Kidney failure is when the kidneys are no longer able to function sufficiently. Water and toxins accumulate and dialysis may be needed.

2. Dialysis artificially removes excess fluid and waste products from the blood.

V. **ASSESSMENT AND MANAGEMENT OF ABDOMINAL, GYNECOLOGICAL, AND GENITOURINARY/RENAL EMERGENCIES**
(See summary of assessment in chapter 12.)

A. Maintain a high index of suspicion for the following:

1. Any patient with abdominal pain associated with fever, bleeding, vomiting, syncope, chest pain, trauma, or signs of shock

2. Any female patient of child-bearing years with abdominal pain

3. Any patient with abdominal pain suggestive of a possible cardiac problem, such as the geriatric, diabetic, and female patients

4. Any patient complaining of severe "tearing" back or flank pain

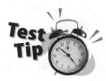

*The end of your training program should **not** be regarded as the end of your preparation for the national certification exam. You shouldn't take the certification exam until you are prepared. Establish a reasonable timetable to prepare for the certification exam.*

PRACTICE QUESTIONS

1. Your patient complains of acute abdominal pain. This means the pain

   A. is severe.

   B. is sharp.

   C. started suddenly.

   D. requires surgery.

2. Your patient complains of abdominal pain that is dull, diffuse, and difficult to localize. This is known as

   A. visceral pain.

   B. parietal pain.

   C. referred pain.

   D. acute pain.

3. Your patient complains of abdominal pain. He states it was diffuse, but is now localized in the right lower abdominal quadrant. The patient denies any trauma or surgeries. Which of the following is most likely?

A. peritonitis

B. appendicitis

C. cholecystitis

D. diverticulitis

4. Your patient complains of abdominal pain. He states he has been experiencing dark, tarry stool and hematochezia. You should suspect

A. GI bleeding.

B. diverticulitis.

C. kidney stones.

D. food poisoning.

5. Which of the following is an infection with associated diarrhea, nausea, and vomiting?

A. gonorrhea

B. food poisoning

C. pancreatitis

D. gastroenteritis

ANSWERS

1. C.

Acute means sudden onset.

2. A.

Visceral abdominal pain is dull, diffuse pain that is difficult to localize. Parietal abdominal pain is severe and localized pain. Referred pain causes pain in an area of the body other than the source. Acute pain has a sudden onset.

3. **B.**

   Appendicitis is most likely. The other choices to not typically present with diffuse pain that eventually localizes to the right lower abdominal quadrant.

4. **A.**

   Dark, tarry stool, hematemesis (vomiting blood), and hematochezia (bloody stool) are signs of gastrointestinal bleeding.

5. **D.**

   Gastroenteritis is an infection with associated diarrhea, nausea, and vomiting. This is a common cause of hypovolemic shock in children.

Behavioral Emergencies

I. INTRODUCTION TO BEHAVIORAL EMERGENCIES

A. Behavioral emergency: abnormal behavior that is unacceptable to patients, family members, or society.

B. Causes of behavioral emergencies can be physiological or psychological.

1. Physiological causes include diabetic emergency; hypoxia; head injury; drugs, alcohol, or toxins; environmental emergencies; and seizures.

2. Psychological causes include

   i. anxiety: unusual level of stress about an event or problem

   ii. bipolar disorder: also known as manic depression; characterized by drastic mood swings

   iii. depression: deep sadness not associated with a specific event

   iv. paranoia: extreme suspicion or distrust about others

   v. phobias: unusual level of fear about specific things

   vi. psychosis: delusional state

   vii. schizophrenia: a state characterized by disorganized speech and thinking

II. SUICIDAL PATIENTS

A. Suicide Facts

1. Females are more likely to attempt suicide, but males are more likely to die as a result of suicide.

2. Suicide attempts usually involve firearms, drugs, or alcohol.

3. Most suicidal patients will give clear signals of their intent.

B. All suicidal gestures should be taken seriously, especially when patients have a clear plan and the means to carry it out.

C. Risk Factors for Suicide

1. History of mental illness, previous suicide attempts, or child abuse

2. Recent diagnosis of serious illness

3. Recent loss of job, family member, or partner

4. Divorced or widowed

III. RISK OF VIOLENCE

A. High-Risk Situations

1. Suicidal patients

2. Patients with agitated delirium

   i. Agitated delirium is characterized by violent, unpredictable behavior, and unusual strength and pain tolerance.

   ii. It is often associated with use of methamphetamine or other central nervous system (CNS) stimulants.

   iii. Agitated delirium patients are at high risk of sudden cardiac arrest.

B. Warning Signs of Potential Violent Behavior

1. Threats or threatening behavior, throwing or striking other objects

2. Pacing or clenched fists

3. Swearing or shouting

IV. PATIENT RESTRAINT

(See chapter 3 for information about patient restraint and use of force.)

Thoroughly document the following for any call requiring patient restraint:

A. The patient's presentation, demeanor, etc.

B. The reason for restraint and method of restraint

C. The time and duration of restraint

D. Continuous monitoring of the patient's level of consciousness (LOC), airway, breathing, and circulator status

E. The patient's pulses, skin color, and temperature in the extremities distal to the restraint devices

F. The role of law enforcement and medical direction

G. The patient's status upon transfer of care

 V. ASSESSMENT AND MANAGEMENT

(See summary of assessment in chapter 12.)

A. Implement the following techniques when managing behavioral patients:

   1. Give patient adequate space, and be prepared for rapid changes in behavior.

   2. Don't block the patient's means of exit or display a judgmental attitude.

   3. Listen actively and don't interrupt.

   4. Don't leave the patient alone. Don't leave your partner alone with the patient.

   5. Don't give ultimatums.

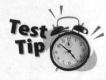

Test Tip

You should prepare for the certification exam as quickly as your schedule will allow. Determine how long it takes you to prepare for half of the content on the certification exam (which equates with the first 19 chapters of this book). If it takes you two weeks to reach the halfway point in your preparations, schedule your exam for two weeks in the future.

Why? Because you know it's an achievable timeframe based on what you have already accomplished, and the second half of your preparations should go even faster than the first. You have already learned some challenging topics, such as airway, assessment, and cardiac and respiratory emergencies. Also, you are now "in the groove" and have momentum.

Working quickly toward the certification exam reduces the amount of information you are "losing" by not attending class any longer.

PRACTICE QUESTIONS

1. Abnormal behavior that is unacceptable to patients, family members, or society considered

    A. a physiological emergency.

    B. a behavioral emergency.

    C. an environmental emergency.

    D. a seizure disorder.

2. Which of the following is a physiological cause of a behavioral emergency?

    A. anxiety

    B. depression

    C. paranoia

    D. alcohol

3. Your patient has been diagnosed with bipolar disorder. This means the patient experiences

   A. a constant, deep sadness.

   B. extreme suspicion of others.

   C. disorganized speech and thinking.

   D. drastic mood swings.

4. Which of the following methods of suicide is most common?

   A. firearms.

   B. hanging.

   C. jumping from heights.

   D. asphyxiation.

5. Which of the following is a known risk factor for suicide?

   A. recent retirement

   B. a recent move

   C. recent divorce

   D. a recent promotion

ANSWERS

1. **B.**

   A behavioral emergency is defined as abnormal behavior that is unacceptable to patients, family members, or society.

2. **D.**

   Physiological causes of behavioral emergencies include diabetic emergency; hypoxia; head injury; drugs, alcohol, or toxins; environmental emergencies; and seizures.

3. **D.**

   Bipolar disorder is characterized by drastic mood swings.

4. A.

Suicide attempts usually involve firearms, drugs, or alcohol.

5. C.

Risk factors for suicide include divorce or loss of spouse.

PART V

TRAUMA AND ENVIRONMENTAL EMERGENCIES

Kinematics of Trauma, Trauma Triage

I. INTRODUCTION TO MECHANISM OF INJURY (MOI) AND KINEMATICS OF TRAUMA

A. The terms "mechanism of injury" (MOI) and "kinematics of trauma" are often used interchangeably to describe the manner in which traumatic injuries occur.

   1. For example, traumatic injuries can be blunt or penetrating, high velocity or low velocity, isolated or multisystem.

   2. Kinetic energy comes from an object in motion.

      i.   Kinetic energy = ½ mass × velocity².

      ii. Note that velocity plays a much bigger role than mass in the energy available to cause trauma.

B. Understanding the MOI helps predict injury patterns and sharpen the EMT's index of suspicion.

   1. Index of suspicion is the ability to determine what types of injuries are possible or likely based on the MOI.

   2. EMS providers don't diagnose; they rule in possibilities based on three key factors: MOI, anatomical findings, and physiological presentation of the patient.

II. INJURY MECHANISMS

A. Motor Vehicle Collisions (MVC)

    1. Types of MVCs

       i. Head-on

          ➤ Occupants can go up and over or down and under the dash.

          ➤ Head, spinal, chest, abdomen, hip, and lower extremity injuries are common. Unrestrained patients are more likely to be ejected.

       ii. Rear impact. Cervical-spine (c-spine) injury due to hyperextension is common.

       iii. Lateral impact (T-bone). Injuries along the side of impact are common.

       iv. Rollover. Injury patterns are difficult to predict. There is a high risk of ejection in rollover MVCs.

       v. Rotational spins. Rotational forces increase the risk of c-spine injury.

    2. Importance of assessing vehicle damage

       i. Assessing the damage to the vehicle helps determine the MOI and the amount of force the patient was exposed to.

       ii. The index of suspicion for serious injury to the patient goes up based on the amount of damage to the vehicle.

    3. Assessing MOI

       i. What did the vehicle hit, and at what speed?

       ii. Where is the damage to the vehicle, and how extensive is it?

       iii. How much intrusion into the patient compartment is there?

       iv. Did airbags deploy? Are the windows intact?

       v. What is the condition of the steering column, steering wheel, and dashboard?

    4. The three collisions

       i. When a vehicle strikes an object, there are three important collisions:

          ➤ First collision: the vehicle strikes an object.

> ➤ Second collision: the passenger strikes interior of the vehicle or safety restraint system (SRS).

> ➤ Third collision: the internal organs strike the internal structures of the body.

    ii. Coup-contrecoup brain injury: brain injury on the opposite side of impact

5. Safety restraint systems (SRS)

    i. The SRS may include a seat belt, shoulder harness, and air bags.

    ii. SRS can reduce deceleration injuries due to second and third collisions and coup-contrecoup injury.

6. Significant MOIs

    i. Rollovers or ejection from the vehicle

    ii. Death of another occupant in the same vehicle

    iii. Pedestrians, cyclists, or motorcyclists struck by vehicle

    iv. Significant damage to the vehicle exterior (above about 18 inches)

    i. Damage intruding into passenger compartment (above about 12 inches)

    vi. Falls greater than 10 feet by a pediatric patient, or any fall with a loss of consciousness

B. Falls. There are three key assessments for fall injuries:

1. The distance fallen: greater than 15 feet or three times patient's height is significant.

2. The surface struck.

3. Body part landed on.

C. Penetrating Trauma

1. Low-velocity projectiles

    i. Examples: knife, pencil, rebar.

    ii. Injury resides along the projectile's path.

2. Medium velocity

    i. Examples: handguns, some rifles.

      ii. Injury pattern is less predictable due to ricochet within body and bullet fragmentation.

  3. High velocity

      i. Example: assault rifles.

      ii. Injury path can be many times larger than projectile due to cavitation (formation of a space within the body along the projectile's path).

D. Blast Injuries

  1. Primary blast injury: injuries due to the pressure wave of the blast

  2. Secondary blast injury: injuries due to flying debris

  3. Tertiary blast injury: injuries caused by being thrown against a stationary object

  4. Miscellaneous blast injuries: injuries due to burns, inhalation injury, etc.

III. TRAUMA TRIAGE

A. Indications for Air Medical Transport.

  1. Extended extrication time, no other ALS providers available, closest trauma centers unavailable, multiple patients requiring transport, traffic conditions delay ground transport, and distance to trauma center greater than 20 miles

B. Hospital Destination

  1. High-priority trauma patients should be seen at an appropriate Level 1 trauma center.

  2. Consult local protocol and medical direction when in doubt about hospital destination.

  3. The national trauma triage protocol is available at the Centers for Disease Control and Prevention website (*http://www.cdc.gov*). Search for "trauma triage." This triage protocol requires determination of the patient's Glasgow Coma Score (see Table 22-1).

Table 22-1 Glasgow Coma Scale (GCS)

Eye opening	Spontaneous	4
	To speech To pain	3
	None	2
		1
Verbal response	Alert and oriented	5
	Confused	4
	Inappropriate	3
	Incomprehensible	2
	None	1
Motor response	Obeys commands	6
	Localizes pain	5
	Withdraws from pain	4
	Abnormal flexion	3
	Abnormal extension	2
	None	1
	Total Score:	Min. 3/Max. 15

Note: A lower GCS score indicates a higher likelihood of brain injury and the need for rapid intervention and transport.

C. Trauma Center Designations

1. Level 1 Trauma Center: capable of handling all types of trauma 24/7. This includes on-site trauma teams, surgical capabilities, trauma intensive care units (ICU), and rehabilitation services

2. Level 2 Trauma Center: capable of stabilizing trauma patients and transferring to a Level 1 trauma center

3. Level 3 and 4 Trauma Centers: Limited services and ability to stabilize trauma patients

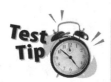
Test Tip

You are past the halfway point! Congratulations. You will likely find many of the remaining chapters a bit easier than those you have already completed; however, they are no less important.

Make sure your flashcards are up to date and you are reviewing at least a few of them every day as often as possible. Repetition is essential! Repetition is essential!

PRACTICE QUESTIONS

1. Which of the following is true regarding a rear-impact motor vehicle collision?

   A. Injuries along the left side of the driver's body are common.

   B. Occupants are likely to go down and under the dash.

   C. Neck injuries due to hyperextension are common.

   D. Injury patterns are unpredictable with a rear-impact collision.

2. The risk of ejection from a motor vehicle collision is highest with

   A. a rotational spin.

   B. a rollover.

   C. a lateral impact.

   D. a head-on collision.

3. Your patient was a passenger in a vehicle that struck a tree. Which of the following is considered the "third collision" based on this mechanism?

   A. The patient's internal organs striking the internal structures of the body.

   B. The vehicle's impact with the tree.

   C. The patient's collision with the seat belts or air bags.

   D. The patient's collision with the interior structures of the vehicle.

4. Which of the following is true regarding vehicle safety restraint systems (SRS)?

   A. A vehicle SRS is not beneficial in a rollover accident.

   B. The SRS eliminates the risk of coup-contrecoup injuries.

   C. The SRS includes a collapsible steering column.

   D. A vehicle SRS can reduce deceleration injuries.

5. Your patient has injuries due to the pressure wave of an explosive device. These injuries are considered

   A. primary blast injuries.

   B. secondary blast injuries.

   C. tertiary blast injuries.

   D. miscellaneous blast injuries.

ANSWERS

1. **C.**

   Cervical spine injuries are common with rear impact MVCs due to hyperextension of the neck.

2. **B.**

   The risk of ejection is highest with an unrestrained occupant in a rollover accident.

3. **A.**

   The first collision occurs when the vehicle strikes the object. The second collision occurs when the passenger strikes the interior of the vehicle or SRS. The third collision occurs when the passenger's internal organs strike the internal structures of the body.

4. **D.**

   A vehicle SRS includes seat belt, shoulder harness, and air bags. The SRS can reduce deceleration injuries due to second and third impacts.

5. **A.**

   Primary blast injuries are due to the pressure wave of the blast.

Bleeding and
Soft Tissue Injuries

Note: Before proceeding with this chapter, review chapter 7 for the anatomy and physiology of the cardiovascular system.

I. BLEEDING

A. Types of Bleeding

1. External bleeding

    i. May be obvious only if the patient is exposed

    ii. More manageable than internal bleeding

2. Internal bleeding

    i. Harder to identify and more difficult to manage than external bleeding

    ii. Signs and symptoms

       ➤ Bruising, hematoma, hematemesis, fractured bones

       ➤ Mechanism of injury (MOI), abdominal distention

       ➤ Bloody or dark, tarry stool or signs and symptoms of shock

B. Sources of Bleeding

1. Arteries: spurting, bright red blood.

2. Veins: steady flow of dark red blood.

3. Capillaries: slow oozing of dark red blood. May be mixed with clearish fluid.

    4. Note that bone fractures can lead to significant arterial and venous bleeding. A liter of blood can be lost from a single femur fracture and even more from a pelvic fracture.

C. Controlling External Hemorrhage

    1. First method

        i.   Apply direct pressure with dry sterile dressing.

        ii. May apply pressure dressing if bleeding is controlled.

    2. Second method. If direct pressure does not control bleeding, apply a tourniquet proximal to the source of bleeding.

    3. If the wound is in a location that does not allow use of a tourniquet, consider use of an approved topical hemostatic agent with continued direct pressure.

    4. Special situations

        i.   Epistaxis (nosebleed)

          ➤ May be due to direct trauma or more serious causes such as hypertension.

          ➤ Blood may be swallowed, increasing the risk of vomiting.

          ➤ Bleeding can usually be controlled by squeezing the nostrils together just below the bridge of the nose for at least 10 minutes.

        ii. Bleeding from nose or ears following head injury

          ➤ May be an indication of skull fracture.

          ➤ Apply a loose dressing, but do not apply direct pressure. This may increase pressure within the skull.

D. Hemorrhagic Shock (See chapter 13.)

E. Pneumatic Anti-Shock Garment (PASG)

    1. Also called the military anti-shock trousers (MAST).

    2. The PASG is a controversial method of treating shock, controlling bleeding, and stabilizing fractures.

    3. The PASG is no longer used in many EMS systems. Consult local protocol and medical direction.

4. Indications: pelvic or lower extremity fractures, shock with systolic pressure below 90 mmHg, severe hypotension (below 60 mmHg)

5. Contraindications: pulmonary edema, pregnancy, penetrating thoracic injury, head injury

6. Do *not*

    i.   delay transport to apply the PASG

    ii. deflate the PASG

    iii. inflate the abdominal compartment without inflating both leg compartments

II. SOFT TISSUE INJURIES (STI)

A. Three Types of Soft Tissue Injuries

1. Open injuries

    i.   Types of open injuries

        ➤ Abrasion: a scrape to the skin due to surface friction

        ➤ Laceration: a jagged cut

        ➤ Penetrating wound: puncture wound

        ➤ Incision: a sharp, clean cut

        ➤ Avulsion: injury caused by a flap of skin being torn partially or completely loose

        ➤ Crush injury: may be open or closed

        ➤ Amputation: when part of the body is severed completely from the rest (See chapter 25 for additional information about amputations.)

    ii. Management of open soft tissue injuries. Treatment is the same as for external bleeding.

        ➤ Apply direct pressure and elevate the injured area.

        ➤ Apply a dressing and bandage.

        ➤ Continue to elevate as needed.

        ➤ Apply a tourniquet for uncontrolled hemorrhage.

    2. Closed injuries

      i.   Types of closed injuries

         ➤ Contusion

         ➤ Hematoma: a collection of blood beneath the skin

         ➤ Crush injury: may be open or closed

      ii. Management of closed soft tissue injuries

         ➤ **RICES**: stands for **R**est, **I**ce, **C**ompression, **E**levation, **S**plinting. This technique reduces pain and swelling.

    3. Burn injuries: see chapter 24.

B. Special Situations

    1. Compartment syndrome

      i.   Compartment syndrome is caused by compression of nerves, blood vessels, and muscle in a closed space within the body.

      ii. The tissue cannot receive adequate blood supply and may die.

      iii. Crush injury can lead to compartment syndrome.

      iv. Severe pain is the primary symptom.

    2. Evisceration

      i.   Open abdominal injury with external organs (usually intestine) protruding

      ii. Management of evisceration

         ➤ Cover with moist sterile dressing.

         ➤ Cover moist dressing with occlusive dressing.

         ➤ Flex legs if possible to reduce abdominal contraction.

         ➤ Treat for shock.

         ➤ This is a high-priority transport.

    3. Impaled objects

      i.   Impaled objects should be stabilized in place.

      ii. There are only two indications for removing an impaled object:

➤ The object creates an airway obstruction or inability to manage the airway, such as an impaled object in the cheek.

➤ The object is in the chest and prevents CPR for a patient in cardiac arrest.

4. Open neck injury. Cover open neck wounds with an occlusive dressing to prevent air embolism.

5. Bite wounds

   i. All bite wounds that break the skin pose a high risk of infection.

   ii. Small animal bites may lead to rabies.

      ➤ Rabies is an acute, deadly viral infection of the central nervous system. If the animal responsible for the bite is not tested for rabies, the patient typically must receive a series of painful injections.

   iii. All bites that break the skin should be evaluated by a physician for infection and the need for a tetanus shot.

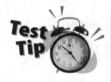

For your exam, be sure you know the five basic interventions for bleeding with signs and symptoms of shock:

1. *Direct pressure for external bleeding*

2. *High-flow oxygen*

3. *Place patient supine*

4. *Prevent heat loss*

5. *High-priority transport*

PRACTICE QUESTIONS

1. Your trauma patient presents with abdominal bruising and distention. Which of the following is most likely?

   A. evisceration

   B. flail segment

   C. hemothorax

   D. internal bleeding

2. You are attempting to control significant external bleeding on your trauma patient. Direct pressure alone is ineffective and the injury is in a location that does not allow use of a tourniquet. You should

   A. use a topical hemostatic agent.

   B. discontinue direct pressure.

   C. place the patient in a seated position.

   D. apply a pressure bandage.

3. Your patient is experiencing epistaxis. This means the patient has

   A. internal bleeding.

   B. dental trauma.

   C. a nosebleed.

   D. blood in the stool.

4. Which of the following soft tissue injuries can be open or closed?

   A. crush injury

   B. avulsion

   C. incision

   D. contusion

5. When should an impaled object be removed?

    A. Never

    B. Always

    C. When it creates an airway obstruction.

    D. When it is difficult to stabilize.

ANSWERS

1. D.

Abdominal bruising and distention are signs of internal bleeding. An evisceration is an open abdominal injury. Flail segment and hemothorax are chest injuries.

2. A.

If bleeding cannot be controlled with direct pressure alone, and a tourniquet cannot be applied, you should use an approved topical hemostatic agent along with direct pressure.

3. C.

Epistaxis is a nosebleed.

4. A.

A crush injury can be open or closed.

5. C.

Impaled objects should be stabilized in place unless they create an airway obstruction or prevent chest compressions for a cardiac arrest patient.

Burn Injuries

I. SEVERITY OF BURN INJURIES

A. The Five Factors of Burn Severity

    1. Depth of burn

        i. Superficial (first-degree) burn

            ➤ Epidermal damage only

            ➤ Painful, red, no blisters

        ii. Partial thickness (second-degree) burn

            ➤ Epidermal and partial dermal injury

            ➤ Painful, blisters present

        iii. Full thickness (third-degree) burn

            ➤ Injury completely through dermal layer

            ➤ Dry, leathery skin; no pain

    2. Amount of body surface area burned

        i. Rule of Nines: totals 100% of body surface area (TBSA)

Rule of Nines

Area	Adults	Children	Infants
Entire head and neck	9%	12%	18%
Anterior chest and abdomen	18%	18%	18%
Posterior chest and abdomen	18%	18%	18%
Entire left leg	18%	16.5%	13.5%
Entire right leg	18%	16.5%	13.5%
Entire left arm	9%	9%	9%
Entire right arm	9%	9%	9%
Groin	1%	1%	1%
Total:	100%	100%	100%

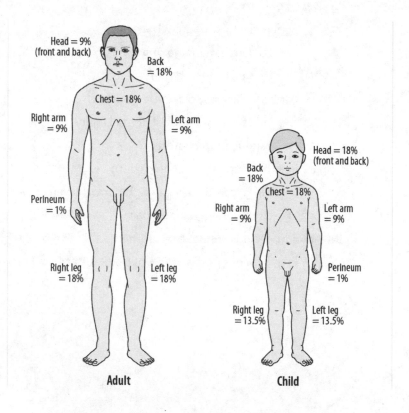

ii. Palm method: palm of patient's hand equals about 1% TBSA

3. Burns to critical areas. The critical areas are the respiratory tract, hands, face, feet, and genitalia.

4. Associated trauma or preexisting medical conditions. Associated trauma, poor health, and certain medications complicate body's ability to handle a burn injury.

5. Age of patient. Under 5 or over 55 years of age are at greater risk.

B. Severe Burn Injuries

1. Burns with respiratory compromise

2. Full-thickness circumferential (all the way around) burns

3. Partial-thickness burns covering more than 30% of TBSA

4. Burns with associated trauma, such as fractures

5. Full-thickness burns to the airway, hands, face, feet, or genitalia

6. Full-thickness burns covering more than 10% of the TBSA

7. All moderate burn criteria for patients under 5 or over 55 years of age

C. Moderate Burn Injuries

1. Full-thickness burns covering 2% to 10% of TBSA

2. Partial-thickness burns covering 15% to 30% of TBSA

3. Superficial burns covering more than 50% TBSA

D. Minor Burn Injuries

1. Full-thickness burns covering less than 2% of TBSA

2. Partial-thickness burns covering less than 15% of TBSA

3. Superficial burns covering less than 50% TBSA.

II. LIFE-THREATENING COMPLICATIONS OF BURN INJURIES

A. The life-threatening complications related to burn injury are sepsis, hypothermia, hypovolemic shock, and airway compromise.

III. THERMAL BURNS

A. Thermal burns are caused by heat, such as from water, steam, or fire.

B. Management of Thermal Burns

1. Stop the burning process with a moist sterile burn sheet until skin is no longer hot to the touch.

2. Replace moist burn sheets with dry sterile burn sheets to reduce risk of hypothermia and infection.

3. Remove clothing that may be trapping heat.

4. Remove jewelry since massive swelling is likely.

5. Treat for shock as needed.

IV. SPECIAL SITUATIONS

A. Inhalation Injury

1. Can occur due to chemical inhalation or if patient inhales hot gases due to fire in a confined space.

2. Signs and symptoms include stridor, dyspnea, coughing, wheezing, facial burns, hoarse voice, airway edema, singed facial hair, or soot in mouth or nose.

B. Electrical Burns

1. Assess scene safety first. Do not attempt to remove patient from an electrical source without proper training.

2. Significant unseen injury may have occurred between entrance and exit points on the body.

3. Electrical burn patients are at high risk of respiratory and cardiac arrest.

4. All electrical injury patients require transport and evaluation by a physician.

C. Chemical Burns

    1. Eyes and respiratory system are at high risk for chemical burn injury.

    2. Assess scene safety first. Do not risk exposure without proper training and personal protective equipment.

    3. If safe to do so

       i.   remove contaminated clothing, jewelry, etc.

       ii. brush off any dry chemical on skin

       iii. irrigate patient with large amounts of water

       iv. avoid contaminating unaffected areas with runoff

    4. Treat as thermal burn.

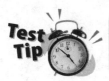

Test Tip

If you plan to use additional publications in preparation for your certification exam, make sure they are based on the current National EMS Education Standards and CPR guidelines. If they are not up-to-date, don't rely on them.

PRACTICE QUESTIONS

1. Your patient has a circumferential burn. This means the burn

    A. goes all the way through the dermis.

    B. covers more than 10% of the body.

    C. goes all the way around.

    D. creates a rounded burn pattern.

2. Your adult patient has a full-thickness burn covering about 5% of his total body surface area. Based on this information, the burn would be considered

    A. minor.

    B. moderate.

    C. severe.

    D. second degree.

3. What is the risk of prolonged application of a wet burn dressing to a significant burn injury?

   A. Hypothermia

   B. Hypertension

   C. Airway compromise

   D. Increased pain

4. Why should you attempt to remove jewelry from your burn patient?

   A. Jewelry must be turned over to investigators.

   B. to reduce the patient's pain

   C. to release trapped heat

   D. Swelling is likely to develop.

5. The palm of the patient's hand equals about

   A. 1% TBSA.

   B. 2% TBSA.

   C. 3% TBSA.

   D. 4% TBSA.

ANSWERS

1. **C.**

   A circumferential burn goes all the way around, such as the arm or chest.

2. **B.**

   A full-thickness burn between 2%–10% TBSA in an adult (excluding other factors) would be considered a moderate burn injury.

3. **A.**

   Prolonged immersion or application of a wet burn dressing increases the risk of hypothermia.

4. **D.**

   Significant swelling is likely following a significant burn. Jewelry may compromise circulation.

5. **A.**

   The palm of the patient's hand equals about 1% of the patient's total body surface area.

Musculoskeletal Injuries

I. TYPES OF INJURIES

A. Fractures

1. Open fracture: a fracture with an associated open soft tissue injury

2. Closed fracture: a fracture where the skin is not broken

3. Signs and symptoms of fracture: pain, swelling, deformity, tenderness, loss of function, possible weak or absent distal pulses and crepitus (the sound or feeling of fractured bone rubbing together)

B. Strain

1. A strain is a stretching injury to a muscle or tendon.

2. Signs and symptoms: pain and tenderness.

3. There is usually little bleeding with a strain, so swelling and discoloration will likely be minimal.

C. Sprain

1. A sprain is in injury to a ligament.

2. Sprains frequently involve the shoulder, knee, or ankle joints.

3. Signs and symptoms

   ➤ Pain and tenderness: immediately

   ➤ Swelling and discoloration: delayed

D. Dislocation

1. A dislocation is the movement of a bone out of its normal position in a joint.

2. The bone may return to its normal position or remain out of joint.

3. Signs and symptoms: pain, deformity, loss of function, possible weak or absent distal pulses.

4. Dislocations often have associated sprains and strains.

E. Potential Limb-Threatening Injuries

1. Any orthopedic injury resulting in loss of circulation distal to the injury is a high-priority injury. The limb is at risk until circulation is restored

2. Signs of orthopedic injury with loss of distal circulation: absence of distal pulses, pale distal to injury, cool distal to injury, delayed capillary refill distal to injury.

F. Potential Life-Threatening Injuries

1. Pelvic fractures

   ➤ One in five hip fracture patients dies within one year of the injury.

   ➤ Hip fracture patients are at risk for hypovolemic shock, embolism, pneumonia, and sepsis.

   ➤ Most hip fractures occur in the geriatric population due to falls.

   ➤ Pelvic binders are commercial splints used in some EMS systems to stabilize pelvic fractures and reduce bleeding.

2. Femur fractures

   ➤ A single femur fracture can cause hypovolemic shock.

   ➤ Femur fracture patients are at an increased risk of pulmonary embolism.

   ➤ Fractures to multiple smaller long bones can combine to cause hypovolemic shock.

3. Amputations

   ➤ Control bleeding.

   ➤ Wrap amputated part in a sterile dressing and place in plastic bag and keep cool.

   ➤ Do not delay transport of a high-priority patient for an amputated part.

II. SPLINTING

A. Correct splinting decreases pain and reduces risk of further injury.

B. Incorrect splinting can

1. increase pain

2. compress blood vessels and compromise circulation

3. inappropriately delay transport of a high-priority patient

C. Rules of Splinting

1. Assess distal pulse, motor, and sensation (PMS) before and after splinting.

   ➤ Pulse: assess pulse distal to injury.

   ➤ Motor: assess patient's ability to move extremity distal to injury.

   ➤ Sensation: assess patient's ability to sense touch distal to injury.

   ➤ Sometimes referred to as "distal neurovascular function" (DNVF).

   ➤ Note: PMS should be regularly reassessed after splint is applied.

2. Immobilize above and below injury.

   ➤ Immobilize injured bone and joints above and below injured bone.

   ➤ Immobilize injured joint and bones above and below injured joint.

3. Attempt to realign deformed injuries with absent distal pulses.

   ➤ If distal pulse is absent, make one attempt to realign with gentle in-line traction (pulling) and reassess distal circulation.

   ➤ If pulse is not restored, treat injury as a high priority.

   ➤ If pain, crepitus, or resistance is encountered, stop and immobilize as is.

4. Do *not* delay transport of a high-priority patient for a non-life-threatening injury.

D. Types of splints: cardboard splints, padded board splints, wire splints, formable splints, pneumatic splints, traction splints, pelvic binders, pillow splints, and triangular bandages

E. Traction Splint

1. There are various kinds of traction splints. Follow local protocol.

2. Indication: closed, midshaft femur fractures.

3. Contraindications

➤ Open femur fracture

➤ Injury to hip, knee, lower leg, or ankle on same side as femur fracture

4. Do *not* delay transport of a high-priority patient to apply a traction splint.

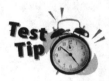

Expose yourself to as many multiple-choice practice questions as possible before your certification exam. Practicing at least 100 questions for each of the five categories on the certification exam is recommended.

Search for sources of practice tests or quizzes that meet the following criteria:

1. Questions are based on current National EMS Education Standards and CPR guidelines.

2. There are a high number of scenario-based questions.

3. Answer sections explain the rationale behind the correct answer.

PRACTICE QUESTIONS

1. Which of the following is considered a potentially limb-threatening injury?

A. Any orthopedic injury with deformity.

B. Any orthopedic injury with significant swelling.

C. Any orthopedic injury with loss of distal circulation.

D. Any orthopedic injury with associated contusions.

2. What is the most common cause of hip fractures in elderly patients?

   A. fall injuries

   B. motor vehicle accidents

   C. pathologic fractures

   D. elderly abuse

3. Which of the following fractures is most likely to increase the risk of pulmonary embolism?

   A. rib fracture

   B. femur fracture

   C. humerus fracture

   D. ulnar fracture

4. Which of the following is the highest priority for a patient with an amputation injury?

   A. Wrap the amputated part in a sterile dressing.

   B. Assure the patient the condition is not permanent.

   C. Control any significant bleeding.

   D. Rapidly reduce the temperature of the amputated part.

5. Your patient has a suspected fracture to the forearm. You should immobilize

   A. the forearm only.

   B. the forearm and wrist.

   C. the humerus, elbow, forearm, wrist, and hand.

   D. the elbow, forearm, and wrist.

ANSWERS

1. **C.**

   Any orthopedic injury with loss of distal pulses should be considered a limb-threatening injury.

2. **A.**

   Fall injuries are the most common cause of hip fractures in elderly patients.

3. **B.**

   Fractures to the femur or pelvis increase the risk of pulmonary embolism.

4. **C.**

   Any potentially life-threatening bleeding must be controlled during the primary assessment and takes priority over wrapping the amputated part. Assuring the patient the injury is temporary or rapidly cooling the amputated part are not appropriate.

5. **D.**

   You should immobilize the injury and the bones or joints immediately proximal and distal to the injury.

Head and Spinal Injuries

I. HEAD INJURIES

A. Head injuries include trauma to the scalp, skull, or brain.

B. Scalp Injuries

1. Scalp injuries can be open or closed.

2. The scalp is highly vascular and bleeds heavily when lacerated.

C. Skull Fractures

1. Skull fractures indicate the potential for injury to the brain.

2. Linear fracture. Most skull fractures are linear fractures and do not present with deformity or depression.

3. Depressed fracture. Depressed skull fractures may be noticeable upon palpation. There is an increased risk of brain injury due to bone being displaced into brain tissue.

4. Basal skull fracture. These fractures occur at the base of the skull. Cerebrospinal fluid may leak from nose or ears. Signs may include Battle's sign (bruising behind the ears) and raccoon eyes (bruising under the eyes).

D. Brain Injuries

1. Concussion

i. A concussion temporarily causes brain function to be disrupted in some manner.

ii. Signs and symptoms typically occur rapidly and gradually improve.

  iii. Signs and symptoms may include altered level of consciousness (LOC) that gradually improves, brief loss of consciousness, nausea, vomiting, irritability, repetitive questioning, vision problems, and amnesia.

   ➤ Anterograde amnesia: can't remember what happened after the injury

   ➤ Retrograde amnesia: can't remember events before the injury

2. Cerebral contusion

  i. Cerebral contusion is often accompanied by edema and/or concussion injury.

  ii. Signs and symptoms of cerebral contusion may include signs of concussion *and* at least one of the following: decreasing mental status, unresponsive, pupillary changes, changes in vital signs, or obvious behavioral abnormalities.

3. Epidural hematoma

  i. Bleeding beneath the skull but above the dura mater

  ii. Typically includes significant arterial bleeding

  iii. Extremely dangerous due to increase in intracranial pressure

  iv. Often accompanied by a temporal skull fracture

  v. Signs and symptoms

   ➤ Patient may experience a brief loss of consciousness, wakes up, then LOC deteriorates.

   ➤ Worsening LOC, headache, seizures, vomiting, posturing, hypertension, bradycardia, changes in respirations, pupillary changes.

4. Subdural hematoma

  i. Bleeding above the brain (beneath the dura mater and above the arachnoid meningeal layer)

  ii. Often caused by venous bleeding following a cerebral contusion

  iii. Signs and symptoms: vomiting, decreasing LOC, pupillary changes, unilateral (one side of the body) weakness or paralysis, hypertension, changes in respirations, headache, and seizures

5. Subarachnoid hemorrhage

   i. Bleeding within the subarachnoid space.

   ii. This type of injury allows blood to enter the cerebrospinal fluid (CSF).

   iii. Can be due to trauma or a ruptured aneurysm.

   iv. Signs often include headache and stiff neck, and neurological impairment such as decreased LOC and seizures.

6. Intracerebral hemorrhage

   i. Bleeding within the brain tissue.

   ii. Patients can deteriorate rapidly.

   iii. High mortality (risk of death) rate.

7. Herniation syndrome

   i. The pressure within the skull is called intracranial pressure (ICP). Herniation is when the brain is compressed due to excessive ICP.

   ii. Remember, the brain is in an enclosed space. There is little extra space to accommodate swelling, bleeding, etc.

   iii. Severe herniation will force the brain down toward the foramen magnum.

   iv. Signs of increased ICP

   ➤ Cushing's response, or Cushing's reflex

   — Hypertension

   — Bradycardia

   — Altered respiratory pattern

   v. Mortality rates are high for ICP patients. In an attempt to temporarily reduce dangerously high ICP, higher ventilation rates may be indicated. Consult local protocol and medical direction.

II. SPINAL INJURIES

A. Mechanism of Injury (MOI) for Spinal Trauma

   1. Flexion: extreme forward (chin-to-chest) movement of head

2. Extension: extreme backward movement of head, such as might occur in a rear-impact accident

3. Compression: compression of head against the body, such as a diving injury

4. Rotation: extreme lateral (side-to-side) movement

5. Distraction: stretching of spinal column and cord, such as a hanging

6. Lateral bending: extreme bending of head to the side (ear to shoulder)

7. Penetrating injury: gunshot wounds, stab wounds, etc.

B. Signs and Symptoms of Spinal Injury

1. Spinal column injury is likely to produce pain or tenderness.

2. Spinal cord injury is likely to produce motor and/or sensory deficits.

   i. Motor deficits: weak or absent grips, pushes, pulls, etc.

   ii. Sensory deficits: inability to feel or sense touch

   iii. Paraplegia: paralysis of the lower extremities

   iv. Quadriplegia: paralysis of all extremities

3. Transected (severed) cord

   i. Paralysis below the level of injury

   ii. Loss of bladder or bowel control

   iii. Possible respiratory arrest if high cervical injury

   iv. Note that patients with trauma to C5 or above are at high risk for respiratory paralysis. Rapid intervention and artificial ventilations may be needed.

4. Neurogenic shock (see chapter 13 for additional information on neurogenic shock)

   i. Any of the above signs and symptoms

   ii. Hypotension without tachycardia

   iii. Priapism (involuntary penile erection)

5. Spinal shock is a condition that can present with any of the above signs and symptoms, but typically resolves within about 24 hours.

C. Spinal Immobilization

  1. Manual immobilization

    i. Manual cervical-spine (c-spine) precautions must be taken immediately if spinal injury is suspected.

    ii. Manual c-spine cannot be released until the patient's head is completely immobilized by other means.

    iii. A cervical collar is *not* a substitute for manual immobilization.

  2. Spinal immobilization techniques

    i. Long spine board

      ➤ Can be used for supine or standing patients

      ➤ Often used if rapid extrication is needed due to potential problems related to airway, breathing, circulation, etc.

    ii. Half spine board

      ➤ Can be used for seated patients, such as during extrication from a vehicle.

      ➤ Use of these devices may require additional time to apply. You must determine if the patient's condition requires more rapid extrication.

III. SPECIAL SITUATIONS

A. Helmets

  1. Athletic helmets

    i. Athletic helmets typically fit well and allow access to the airway without removing the entire helmet.

    ii. The face mask or guard can usually be unsnapped, unscrewed, or cut. This should be done prior to transport.

    iii. Immobilization of the helmet typically secures the head and cervical spine also.

  2. Motorcycle helmets

    i. Motorcycle helmets may not be a good fit for the patient, so immobilization of the helmet may not immobilize the head and cervical spine.

        ii.   Depending on the style, motorcycle helmets may prevent the EMT from accessing the airway.

    3. In most cases, the patient should be immobilized with the helmet in place.

    4. The helmet should be removed if

        i.   the EMT is unable to access the airway

        ii.   the helmet is too large and does not allow spinal immobilization

B. Pediatric Patients

    1. Pad behind shoulders prior to immobilization.

        i.   Infants and children have a larger head in proportion to their body. When supine, the head will be pushed forward preventing neutral, in-line spinal immobilization.

        ii.   Padding behind the shoulders will help maintain neutral, in-line spinal immobilization.

    2. Car seats. Do *not* use a car seat that has been involved in a motor vehicle collision.

C. The Glasgow Coma Scale (GCS) can help classify the severity of a head injury. (See chapter 22.)

        i.   Mild: a GCS between 13 and 15

        ii.   Moderate: a GCS between 8 and 12

        iii.   Severe: a GCS less than 8

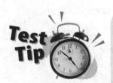

Test Tip

Remember, the purpose of exposing yourself to practice questions is to identify content you need to study before the test. It is not *to memorize the answers to specific questions.*

As you review practice questions, pay particular attention to those you get wrong. Determine if the questions reveal specific topics you need to review further before taking the certification exam. If so, make a flashcard!

PRACTICE QUESTIONS

1. Battle's sign and raccoon's eyes are signs of a

   A. basal skull fracture.

   B. temporal fracture.

   C. linear fracture.

   D. concussion injury.

2. You are assessing a patient who was struck in the head by a baseball. Your patient is having trouble remembering events prior to the injury. This is known as

   A. anterograde amnesia.

   B. retrograde amnesia.

   C. diffuse amnesia

   D. concussive amnesia.

3. Your patient was struck in the head by a baseball. Witnesses state he experienced a brief loss of consciousness and then woke up. You note his LOC is now deteriorating. You should be most concerned about

   A. an epidural hematoma.

   B. a concussion.

   C. an orbital fracture.

   D. Battle's sign.

4. Herniation syndrome is the result of

   A. an open skull fracture.

   B. increased intracranial pressure.

   C. decreased intracranial pressure.

   D. an elevated systolic blood pressure.

5. Which of the following signs are known as Cushing's response?

   A. Hypotension, tachycardia, bradypnea

   B. Hypertension, tachycardia, altered respiratory pattern

   C. Hypotension, bradycardia, bradypnea

   D. Hypertension, bradycardia, altered respiratory pattern

ANSWERS

1. A.

Battle's sign (bruising behind the ears) and raccoon's eyes (bruising under the eyes) are signs of a possible basal skull fracture.

2. B.

Retrograde amnesia is an inability to remember events before the injury. Anterograde amnesia is an inability to remember events after the injury.

3. A.

A brief loss of consciousness following a blow to the head indicates a possible epidural hematoma. This is a more serious concern than a concussion. Battle's sign is a physical finding, not a type of injury.

4. B.

Herniation syndrome is when the brain is physically compressed due to excessive intracranial pressure (pressure within the skull).

5. D.

Cushing's response indicates increased ICP and presents with hypertension, bradycardia, and an altered respiratory pattern.

Chest and Abdominal Trauma

I. CHEST INJURIES

A. Chest injuries result from blunt or penetrating trauma.

B. Signs and symptoms of chest injuries include pain or tenderness, crepitus, bruising or penetrating injury to anterior, lateral, or posterior thorax, paradoxical motion: part of the chest appears to move in opposite direction of the rest of the thoracic cage, respiratory distress, hemoptysis (coughing up blood), jugular venous distention (JVD), hypoxia, abnormal lung sounds, and shock.

C. Types of Chest Injuries

1. Pneumothorax

   i. Pneumothorax is the accumulation of air in the pleural space. This can compress lung space, prevent gas exchange, and lead to hypoxia.

   ii. Can be due to trauma or nontraumatic injury to lung tissue.

   iii. Lung sounds may be diminished or absent over injured area.

2. Tension pneumothorax

   i. A tension pneumothorax causes a progressive collapsing of lung tissue.

   ii. The entire lung and great vessels can be compressed to the other side of the chest. Lung sounds will be absent over the affected area.

   iii. The patient will develop severe respiratory distress and eventually respiratory failure. Compression of the great vessels can restrict blood flow, leading to shock and death.

iv. Tracheal deviation toward the *unaffected* side is a late and ominous sign.

3. Sucking chest wound (also called an open pneumothorax)

   i. If an open chest injury penetrates the pleural space, it can draw air during inhalation.

   ii. Penetrating thoracic injuries should be covered with a three-sided occlusive dressing to prevent air from entering the chest cavity.

4. Hemothorax. A hemothorax is bleeding into the pleural space. Watch for signs and symptoms of shock. Surgery is frequently required to control bleeding.

5. Cardiac tamponade (also known as pericardial tamponade)

   i. Cardiac tamponade occurs when blood or other fluid accumulates in the pericardial sac and compresses the heart.

   ii. Cardiac function can be severely compromised, leading to circulatory collapse.

   iii. Beck's triad (indicative of cardiac tamponade)

       ➤ JVD

       ➤ Muffled heart sounds

       ➤ Narrowing pulse pressure (difference between systolic and diastolic pressures)

6. Clavicle and rib fractures

   i. Clavicle and rib fractures are common and should not be dismissed.

   ii. Clavicle and rib fractures can be associated with pneumothorax.

   iii. A fracture to one of the first several ribs indicates a serious mechanism of injury. Additional injuries should be suspected.

   iv. Patient may present with subcutaneous emphysema. Subcutaneous emphysema is a "crackling" sensation upon palpation due to air escaping into the fatty tissue.

7. Flail chest

    i.   Occurs when a portion of the thorax becomes separated from the rest of the thorax.

    ii.   Caused by the fracture of at least two consecutive ribs in two or more places. It can also occur if the sternum becomes separated from the rib cage.

    iii.   The patient may exhibit paradoxical motion of the separated portion of the chest wall. Paradoxical motion occurs when a portion of the chest wall appears to move in the opposite direction of the rest of the thoracic cage.

    iv.   Patients with a suspected flail chest and inadequate breathing should be ventilated with a BVM and high flow oxygen. Ensuring adequate ventilation is a higher priority than applying a bulky dressing to the thorax.

II. ABDOMINAL INJURIES

A. Solid organs bleed when injured. The primary risk to the patient is hemorrhagic shock. Solid organs include the spleen, liver, kidneys, and pancreas.

B. Hollow organs can spill their contents when injured. The primary risk to the patient is infection. Hollow organs include the stomach, intestines, and urinary bladder.

C. Signs and symptoms of abdominal injury include pain or tenderness; distention; bruising; guarding (patient stiffens abdominal muscles); Kehr's sign: referred pain in the shoulder caused by blood in the peritoneal cavity; and signs and symptoms of shock.

D. See chapter 23 for additional information about open abdominal injuries.

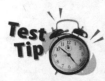

Here are just a couple things from this chapter you must know before the certification exam. Get your flashcards ready!

1. *What is the most important intervention for a flail chest with respiratory compromise?*

2. *What type of dressing should be applied to a sucking chest wound?*

3. *Know Cushing's response and what it indicates.*

4. *Know Beck's triad and what it indicates.*

Answers:

1. *Positive pressure ventilation and oxygen*

2. *A three-sided occlusive dressing*

3. *Hypertension, bradycardia, altered respiratory pattern. Indicates possible closed head injury with increased ICP.*

4. *JVD, muffled heart tones, narrowing pulse pressure. Indicates possible pericardial tamponade.*

PRACTICE QUESTIONS

1. A progressive collapsing of lung tissue due to accumulation of air in the thorax is known as a

    A. simple pneumothorax.

    B. hemothorax.

    C. pulmonary embolism.

    D. tension pneumothorax.

2. An open pneumothorax is also known as a

    A. sucking chest wound.

    B. flail chest.

    C. hemothorax.

    D. pulmonary embolism.

3. Beck's triad indicates
   A. a closed head injury.
   B. a flail chest.
   C. cardiac tamponade.
   D. pulmonary embolism.

4. You suspect your patient has a flail chest. The patient presents with severe respiratory distress. You should immediately
   A. apply oxygen with a nonrebreather mask.
   B. initiate BVM ventilations.
   C. place a bulky dressing over the chest.
   D. obtain a pulse oximetry reading.

5. Which of the following is the correct management of a sucking chest wound?
   A. Apply a three-sided occlusive dressing.
   B. Apply a bulky dressing.
   C. Apply a sterile gauze pad.
   D. Apply an occlusive dressing secured on all sides.

ANSWERS

1. **D.**

   A tension pneumothorax (pneumo = air) is a progressive collapsing of the lung due to the accumulation of air in the pleural space.

2. **A.**

   An open pneumothorax is also called a sucking chest wound.

3. **C.**

   Beck's triad is JVD, muffled heart tones, and narrowing pulse pressure. These findings indicate a cardiac tamponade (also known as pericardial tamponade).

4. **B.**

The priority for any patient with severe respiratory distress is to ensure adequate ventilations. BVM ventilations should be initiated immediately.

5. **A.**

The correct management of a sucking chest wound is a three-sided occlusive dressing.

Eye, Face, and Neck Trauma

I. EYE INJURIES

A. Foreign Objects

1. Non-penetrating foreign objects on the sclera are often easily removed by irrigating the eye.

2. Foreign objects in any other part of the eye should be removed by a physician.

3. Note that some EMS systems allow irrigation of the eyes only for chemical burns. Consult local protocol and medical direction.

B. Corneal Abrasion

1. Direct trauma and foreign objects can cause a corneal abrasion.

2. The cornea is the transparent covering over the iris and pupil.

3. Symptoms include pain, tearing, and the sensation of something in the eye.

C. Orbital Fracture

1. Orbital fractures indicate a significant mechanism of injury (MOI).

2. Consider possibility of associated spinal trauma.

3. Symptoms include visual disturbances, double vision, deformity around the orbit, loss of sensation around the orbit, and the inability to move eye in an upward gaze.

4. Suspected orbital fractures require physician evaluation.

D. Chemical Burns

1. Chemicals in the eye require immediate and continuous irrigation.

    2. Avoid irrigating chemicals from one eye into the other.

  E. Impaled Objects

    1. Do *not* remove impaled objects from the eye.

    2. Stabilize object in place.

    3. Keep both eyes closed to prevent passive movement of impaled object.

  F. Contact Lenses

    1. Procedure for removing contact lenses varies depending on the type of contacts. Removal may be more easily accomplished with a specially designed moistened suction cup.

    2. Consult local protocol and medical direction.

II. FACE INJURIES

  A. Loss of Tooth (dental avulsion)

    1. Control any bleeding to reduce risk of swallowing blood and vomiting.

    2. Rinse tooth with saline and transport in saline-soaked gauze.

  B. Impaled Object in the Cheek

    1. Stabilize the object in place unless it interferes with airway management.

    2. Remove object only if it causes an airway obstruction or interferes with ability to manage airway.

  C. Nosebleed (See chapter 23.)

  D. Ear Injuries

    1. Treat as a soft tissue injury.

    2. Assess MOI for other possible injuries.

III. **NECK INJURIES**

A. Priorities for neck injuries are as follows:

1. Secure the airway.

2. Control life-threatening bleeding.

3. Apply occlusive dressing to large open-neck injury to reduce risk of air embolism.

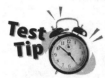

The following concepts were mentioned previously but are important enough to re-emphasize:

When studying or making flashcards, do not focus on memorizing specific questions. Focus on learning important material so you can handle any question over that same material on the certification exam.

Think of practice questions as a tool for searching out content you want to learn before the certification exam. Not every question should result in another flashcard. Focus on the questions you get wrong that identify specific topics you need to learn before the test.

PRACTICE QUESTIONS

1. How should most cases of non-penetrating foreign objects on the sclera be managed?

   A. Bandage both eyes.

   B. Use a cotton swab to remove the object.

   C. Irrigate the eye.

   D. Have the patient blink rapidly.

2. Your patient experienced facial trauma and now complains of double vision. You note deformity around the left orbit. You should suspect a(n)

   A. orbital fracture.

   B. corneal abrasion.

   C. mandibular injury.

   D. mastoid fracture.

3. Which of the following helps reduce passive movement of an impaled object in the eye?

   A. Place the patient supine.

   B. Keep the uninjured eye open.

   C. Keep both eyes closed.

   D. Remove the impaled object.

4. Your patient has a tooth knocked out during a fight. You should

   A. place the tooth in a plastic bag.

   B. wrap the tooth in an occlusive dressing.

   C. wrap the tooth in a dry, sterile dressing.

   D. place the tooth in saline-soaked gauze.

5. What should be done to reduce the risk of air embolism for a large open neck wound?

   A. Apply a tourniquet.

   B. Apply an occlusive dressing.

   C. Place the patient seated upright.

   D. Place gentle pressure on both sides of the neck.

ANSWERS

1. **C.**

   Non-penetrating foreign objects on the sclera are often easily removed by irrigating the eye.

2. **A.**

   The presentation is consistent with an orbital fracture. The mandible is the jaw and the mastoid is behind the ears.

3. **C.**

   Keep both eyes closed to reduce passive movement (eyes work together, not independently). Do NOT remove impaled objects in the eye.

4. **D.**

   Rinse an avulsed tooth with saline and transport in saline-soaked gauze.

5. **B.**

   Apply an occlusive dressing to a large open neck wound to reduce the risk of air embolism.

Environmental Emergencies

I. PATIENT FACTORS INFLUENCING HEAT AND COLD EMERGENCIES

A. Age. The very young and very old will likely develop environmental emergencies more rapidly.

B. General Health and Nutrition. Those in good health, adequately nourished, and hydrated are better able to maintain homeostasis.

C. Environmental Conditions. Temperature, humidity, and wind can help or hurt the body's ability to protect itself from environmental emergencies.

D. Medications and Alcohol. Medications and alcohol can hinder the body's ability to regulate body temperature.

II. COLD EMERGENCIES

A. Two important systemic effects of cold on the body are vasoconstriction (to conserve heat) and an eventual slowing of the metabolic rate.

B. The body loses heat in five basic ways.

1. Conduction: direct transfer of heat through contact with a colder structure. Example: bare feet on a cold floor.

2. Convection: loss of heat to passing air. Example: standing in a cold breeze.

3. Evaporation: loss of heat through evaporation of water from the skin. Example: getting out of the pool or shower.

4. Respiration: in a cold environment, exhaled air has been warmed within the body. That heat is lost on exhalation.

5. Radiation: transfer of radiant heat. Example: entering a walk-in freezer.

C. Hypothermia

1. Hypothermia is a systemic cold emergency. It affects the entire body, not just an isolated area.

2. Hypothermia develops when the body's core temperature falls below that needed to maintain homeostasis.

3. Signs and symptoms of hypothermia

   i. Note that the signs and symptoms of hypothermia get progressively more severe as the core body temperature falls.

   ii. Skin

     ➤ Hypothermic patients will develop cold skin even at their core. Assess by feeling the torso, not the extremities or forehead.

     ➤ Pale and/or cyanosis.

   iii. Shivering

     ➤ Shivering occurs early and helps increase body heat.

     ➤ It ceases with extreme hypothermia.

   iv. Loss of coordination

     ➤ Muscles begin to stiffen.

     ➤ Patient has difficulty speaking.

   v. Altered level of consciousness (LOC)

     ➤ LOC can range from confused to coma in severe hypothermia.

     ➤ As mentation falters, patients may lose survival instincts and leave shelter or remove clothing.

   vi. Vitals

     ➤ Bradycardia, bradypnea, and hypotension.

     ➤ Vitals can be so depressed, the patient appears to be in cardiac arrest even when they are not.

vii. Severe untreated hypothermia will eventually lead to coma, cardiac arrest, and death.

4. Management of hypothermia

   i. Manage life-threatening conditions.

      ➤ Pulse check should be extended to determine if patient is in cardiac arrest or severely bradycardic.

      ➤ Consult local protocol regarding use of automatic external defibrillator (AED) for hypothermic patients.

   ii. Remove patient from cold environment.

   iii. Remove wet clothing; prevent further heat loss.

      ➤ Prehospital rewarming is often limited to passive rewarming measures only (such as blankets). Consult local protocol and medical direction.

      ➤ Rewarming too rapidly can cause ventricular fibrillation.

D. Local Cold Emergencies

   1. Those parts of the body exposed to the environment, such as hands, feet, nose, and ears, are at most risk for local cold emergencies.

   2. Frostnip

      i. Frostnip (also called chilblains) develops when body parts get very cold but are not yet frozen.

      ii. Signs and symptoms include pale and cold skin, and loss of sensation in affected areas.

   3. Trench foot. Also called immersion foot, trench foot can develop when the feet have prolonged exposure to cold and water.

   4. Frostbite

      i. Frostbite is the most dangerous local cold emergency.

      ii. The tissue is frozen, which frequently leads to permanent damage.

      iii. Frostbite can lead to gangrene (tissue death), which can lead to systemic infection and death if untreated.

      iv. Signs and symptoms

         ➤ Hard, frozen tissue

> ➤ Possible blistering

> ➤ Possible mottling

5. Management of local cold emergencies

   i.   Remove patient from cold environment.

   ii.   Remove wet clothing.

   iii.   Protect affected areas from further injury.

   iv.   Remove any jewelry.

   v.   Bandage, splint affected areas.

   vi.   Keep patient immobile.

   vii.   Do *not* rub affected areas.

   viii.   Do *not* apply direct heat unless authorized by medical direction.

III. HEAT EMERGENCIES

A. Two important systemic effects of heat on the body are vasodilation (to shed excess heat) and an increase in metabolic rate.

B. Heat Cramps

1. Heat cramps are a local heat emergency.

2. Heat cramps typically occur during prolonged exertion and are likely caused by an electrolyte imbalance and dehydration.

3. Management of heat cramps includes rest, rehydration, and restoration of electrolytes.

C. Heat Exhaustion

1. Heat exhaustion is a systemic heat emergency and occurs frequently.

2. Heat exhaustion is caused by a combination of heat exposure and hypovolemia.

3. Signs and symptoms of heat exhaustion

   i.   History of exertion in a warm environment

   ii.   Dizziness, weakness

  iii. Nausea, vomiting

  iv. Headache

  v. Possible muscle and abdominal cramps

  vi. Thirst

  vii. Tachycardia

  viii. Possible positive changes in orthostatic vitals (See chapter 10 for information on orthostatic vitals.)

D. Heatstroke

  1. Heatstroke is an uncommon, extremely dangerous systemic heat emergency.

  2. The body loses the ability to regulate body heat. Body temperature rises rapidly and will lead to death if left untreated.

  3. Heatstroke can develop due to exertion, or from passive exposure to a hot environment (for example, a home without air-conditioning during a heat spell or a child left in a hot car).

  4. Signs and symptoms of heatstroke

   i. Similar to those of heat exhaustion.

   ii. Altered or decreased LOC.

   iii. Skin may be hot and dry or wet.

   iv. Seizures.

E. Management of Systemic Heat Emergencies

  1. Move patient to a cooler environment.

  2. If patient is completely alert, water can be administered.

  3. If heatstroke is suspected, cooling measures must be rapid and aggressive.

   i. Expose patient to improve dissipation of heat.

   ii. Cool patient with water, wet towels, cold packs, etc.

   iii. Cold packs are best applied to groin, neck, armpits.

   iv. Rapid transport is indicated.

   v. Prepare for vomiting and/or seizures.

IV. **MISCELLANEOUS ENVIRONMENTAL EMERGENCIES**

A. Scene safety is the top priority during all environmental emergencies.

B. Drowning and Diving Injuries

1. Drowning patients are at risk for aspiration, cardiac arrest, trauma, cervical-spine (c-spine) injury, and hypothermia.

2. Do not attempt water rescue without proper training.

3. Consider possible c-spine injury if unsure how patient entered the water.

4. Consult medical direction regarding possible transport to decompression chamber.

C. Lightning Injuries

1. Treat as a trauma patient.

2. Victims in cardiac arrest due to lightning strikes may be savable with rapid ventilatory support, CPR, and defibrillation with an AED.

3. Manage respiratory arrest and cardiac arrest aggressively. Apply AED rapidly.

D. Bites and Stings

1. Monitor the patient's airway, breathing, circulatory status, and LOC.

2. Clean the wound.

3. Consider applying a cold pack.

4. If the patient demonstrates any systemic complications, transport rapidly.

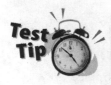

By now, you should have two stacks of flashcards: those you know well, and those you don't know yet. You should be able to memorize at least five new flashcards per day. Remember to regularly review those you have already memorized to make sure you retain the information.

Fear not! You will eventually run out of content for new flashcards and gain quickly on those you still need to learn.

PRACTICE QUESTIONS

1. Your environmental patient is experiencing peripheral vasoconstriction and a slowing metabolic rate. The patient is most likely experiencing a

   A. local heat emergency.

   B. systemic heat emergency.

   C. local cold emergency.

   D. systemic cold emergency.

2. Your patient was found wandering outside on a cold, calm night. The patient was wearing only shorts and shoes. Which of the following would most likely cause this patient to become hypothermic?

   A. conduction

   B. convection

   C. evaporation

   D. radiation

3. Rewarming a hypothermic patient too rapidly can lead to

   A. ventricular fibrillation.

   B. bradycardia.

   C. tachypnea.

   D. hyperventilation syndrome.

4. Which of the following is a common systemic heat emergency caused by a combination of heat exposure and hypovolemia?

   A. heat stroke

   B. heat exhaustion

   C. heat cramps

   D. hypertensive crisis

5. If you suspect your patient is experiencing heat stroke, your cooling measures must be

   A. slow and cautious.

   B. monitored by ALS personnel.

   C. delayed until arrival at the hospital.

   D. rapid and aggressive.

ANSWERS

1. **D.**

   Vasoconstriction and a slowing metabolic rate are typically the result of a systemic cold emergency. A systemic heat emergency would likely cause vasodilation and an increased metabolic rate.

2. **D.**

   Radiation is the transfer of radiant heat, in this case from the patient to the cold environment.

3. **A.**

   Rewarming a hypothermic patient too rapidly can increase the risk of ventricular fibrillation.

4. **B.**

   Heat exhaustion is a common systemic heat emergency caused by heat exposure and hypovolemia. Heat stroke is not a common heat emergency. Heat cramps are a local heat emergency. Hypertensive crisis is not a heat emergency.

5. **D.**

   Cooling measures for a suspected heat stroke patient must be rapid and aggressive to minimize the risk of further brain damage.

PART VI

SPECIAL PATIENT POPULATIONS

Childbirth, Obstetrical Emergencies, Newborn Care

I. GESTATIONAL DEVELOPMENT

A. A full-term pregnancy lasts about 9 months or 40 weeks.

B. Pregnancy is divided into three stages (trimesters).

1. First trimester: first three months of pregnancy

2. Second trimester: middle three months of pregnancy

3. Third trimester: last three months of pregnancy

II. ANATOMICAL AND PHYSIOLOGICAL CHANGES IN PREGNANCY

A. Reproductive Changes

1. The uterus requires a much larger blood supply during pregnancy.

2. The enlarging uterus displaces other internal structures.

B. Respiratory Changes

1. Respiratory rate increases slightly, but oxygen demand increases significantly.

2. In third trimester, the diaphragm frequently is compressed by the enlarging uterus.

3. The pregnant patient is at risk for developing hypoxia rapidly.

C. Cardiovascular Changes

1. Cardiac workload increases, resulting in faster resting heart rate.

2. Blood volume increases, but plasma increase is greater. This leads to relative anemia.

3. Signs and symptoms of shock are masked during pregnancy.

4. Postural hypotension is common, increasing the risk of syncope.

D. Gastrointestinal and Urinary Changes

1. The pregnant patient typically has undigested food in the stomach.

2. Pregnancy increases the risk of nausea and vomiting.

3. Pregnancy increases urinary frequency, and the pregnant patient is at risk of bladder injury due to displacement.

E. Musculoskeletal Changes.

1. The woman's center of gravity changes, increasing the risk of a fall injury.

III. OBSTETRICAL EMERGENCIES

A. Hemorrhage

1. Hemorrhagic shock can develop quickly in the pregnant patient.

2. Signs and symptoms may not be evident until the pregnant patient is in severe shock.

3. Bleeding can occur with little or no external blood loss.

4. Bleeding may be painful or painless.

5. Several conditions can lead to severe bleeding, including placenta previa, abruptio placenta, ectopic pregnancy, uterine rupture, and spontaneous abortion.

B. Placenta Previa

1. Placenta previa is a common cause of bleeding in the third trimester.

2. Placenta previa occurs when the placenta attaches to the uterus over the cervical opening.

3. As the cervix dilates, the placenta is torn and bleeds.

4. Classic presentation is painless vaginal bleeding in the third trimester.

5. Assess for signs and symptoms of shock.

C. Abruptio Placenta

1. Abruptio placenta is the premature separation of the placenta from the uterine wall leading to bleeding.

2. Oxygen and nutrient delivery to fetus is compromised.

3. Maternal blood loss can be severe.

4. The fetus will not survive a complete abruption.

5. Classic presentation is painful vaginal bleeding in the third trimester.

6. Assess for signs and symptoms of shock.

D. Ectopic Pregnancy

1. Ectopic pregnancy occurs when the egg is implanted outside of the uterus, usually in the fallopian tube.

2. Ectopic pregnancy can lead to rupture and severe bleeding.

3. Classic presentation is severe abdominal pain with or without vaginal bleeding.

4. Assess for signs and symptoms of shock.

E. Uterine Rupture

1. The uterus thins as it grows, increasing the risk of rupture.

2. Danger to mother and fetus is high.

3. Classic presentation is abdominal pain and vaginal bleeding.

F. Spontaneous Abortion

1. Spontaneous abortion (miscarriage) is delivery of the fetus before it is capable of surviving. This is prior to about the 20th to 22nd week of pregnancy.

2. Classic presentation includes cramping, lower abdominal pain, vaginal bleeding, and passage of tissue or clots.

3. Assess for signs and symptoms of shock.

G. Seizures

   1. Pregnancy can increase the risk of seizures in the mother.

   2. Management of seizures during pregnancy

      i. Treat as regular seizures (see chapter 16).

      ii. Place patient on left side.

      iii. Minimize exposure to stimulus such as lights, noise, and movement.

H. Preeclampsia and Eclampsia

   1. Preeclampsia (toxemia of pregnancy)

      i. Preeclampsia typically occurs in the third trimester.

      ii. The cause is not completely understood.

      iii. Signs and symptoms include sudden weight gain, visual disturbances; sudden swelling of the face, hands, or feet; headache; and hypertension.

   2. Eclampsia

      i. Eclampsia occurs when the mother seizes following preeclampsia.

      ii. Eclampsia is a life-threatening condition for mother and fetus.

I. Pregnancy-Induced Hypertension (PIH)

   1. PIH is defined as a blood pressure in a pregnant patient above 140/90 at least twice at six hours apart.

   2. PIH presents with the same signs and symptoms as preeclampsia.

J. Supine Hypotensive Syndrome

   1. Supine hypotensive syndrome occurs when the fetus compresses the inferior vena cava. This can cause a severe drop in blood pressure.

   2. This syndrome typically occurs in the later stages of pregnancy when the mother is supine.

   3. Signs and symptoms include dizziness, hypotension, pale skin, and altered level of consciousness (LOC).

   4. Management of supine hypotensive syndrome must include keeping the fetus off the inferior vena cava.

5. Do *not* place the patient in a supine position. Instead,

    i.   place the patient in a seated position

    ii.   place patient on her left or right side

    iii.   if patient is supine, elevate right hip or tilt backboard

IV. TRAUMA AND PREGNANCY

A. Pregnant patients are at an increased risk of trauma.

1. Increased risk of fall injuries

2. Increased risk of domestic abuse

B. Any injury to the mother can pose significant risk to the fetus.

1. The physiological changes that occur during pregnancy mask the usual signs and symptoms of shock.

2. Maintain an extremely high index of suspicion for any pregnant patient who experiences trauma, even in the absence of obvious signs and symptoms of injury, shock, or hypoxia.

3. The fetus may be in serious jeopardy even if the mother appears uninjured.

C. Management of the Pregnant Trauma Patient

1. Conduct a thorough assessment.

2. Determine specifics about the pregnancy during the SAMPLE history.

3. Do *not* place the pregnant patient supine due to the risk of supine hypotensive syndrome.

4. Administer high-flow oxygen.

5. Transport to an appropriate facility. If unsure, request ALS or contact medical direction.

V. PATIENT HISTORY

A. Are you pregnant? If so, how far along? Due date?

B. How many pregnancies have you had (gravida)? How many live births (para)? *Note:* Multiple births count as one birth event.

C. Are you currently receiving prenatal care?

D. Have you experienced any complications with current or previous pregnancies?

E. Are you expecting multiple births, such as twins?

F. Are you experiencing any abdominal pain or vaginal bleeding?

VI. LABOR AND DELIVERY

A. Stages of Labor

1. First stage

i. Begins with the onset of contractions and ends with full cervical dilation.

ii. The cervix is fully dilated at 10 cm, allowing the infant's head to enter the birth canal.

iii. Contractions initially occur at widespread intervals and become more severe and closer together over time.

iv. The mucus plug that seals the uterine opening passes.

v. The amniotic sac may rupture spontaneously.

vi. Stage one typically lasts longer for first-time pregnancies.

2. Second stage

i. Begins with full cervical dilation and ends with delivery of the baby.

ii. Contractions are close together.

iii. Mother feels intense pressure and the urge to push.

3. Third stage

i. Begins once baby is delivered and ends with delivery of the placenta.

ii. Placenta typically delivers within 30 minutes after delivery of the baby.

iii. There will be an increase in vaginal bleeding shortly before the placenta delivers, and the mother will feel the urge to push again.

B. Transport or Deliver on Scene

1. Transport the mother to the hospital for delivery whenever possible. If delivery appears imminent, you should prepare to deliver on scene.

2. Consult medical direction to assist with decision.

3. The following are indications of possible imminent delivery:

   i.   The mother has strong, frequent contractions under two minutes apart with little break between contractions.

      ➤ *Note:* Contractions are timed from the beginning of one contraction to the beginning of the next contraction.

   ii. The abdomen is rigid during contractions.

   iii. The mother feels the urge to push.

   iv. The mother may report passage of the mucus plug and/or uterine rupture.

   v.   Crowning

      ➤ Crowning is the appearance of the baby's head in the birth canal.

      ➤ Assess for crowning if you suspect imminent delivery.

C. Preparing for Delivery

1. Prepare obstetrical (OB) kit.

2. Position the mother—*not* supine: semi-reclined, knees drawn, bottom slightly elevated, feet planted.

3. Expose vaginal opening, assess for crowning, and apply clean sheets around birth area.

4. Tear the amniotic sac if it has not already ruptured.

5. Apply gentle pressure to infant's skull (avoid fontanelles) as head presents in birth canal.

6. As the head delivers, check if the cord is wrapped around the baby's neck (nuchal cord). If the cord is around the neck, gently remove it from around the neck. Be extremely cautious about clamping and cutting the cord, especially if multiple births are a possibility.

7. Suction fluid from baby's mouth and nose once the head clears the birth canal.

8. Guide the presenting shoulder gently up. Once it clears, gently guide the baby downward to help clear the other shoulder. Never pull on the baby.

9. Support the baby upon delivery.

10. Begin assessment and management of the newborn.

11. Clamp and cut the cord once it stops pulsating.

12. Prepare for delivery of the placenta. Gently guide placental delivery, but never pull.

13. Uterine massage and breastfeeding can help reduce postpartum hemorrhage.

14. Transport mother, baby, and placenta.

VII. NEWBORN (NEONATAL) CARE

A. Immediately upon delivery, place on clean, dry sheets or towels.

B. Dry baby, including the head, and immediately replace wet linen with dry.

C. Warm the baby, including the head. Placing the baby on the mother's abdomen will provide a radiant heat source.

D. Suction the baby's mouth first, then nose.

E. If the baby is not active and crying, attempt tactile stimulation by rubbing the baby's back or tapping the soles of the feet.

F. Assess respirations. If the baby is not breathing adequately, begin ventilations (40 to 60 per minute) with an appropriately sized bag and mask for 30 seconds with high-flow oxygen. Do *not* overinflate the newborn's chest.

G. Assess heart rate.

1. Heart rate below 60 beats per minute

i. Begin chest compressions and ventilations at a 3:1 ratio.

ii. Reassess every 30 seconds.

2. Heart rate above 60 but below 100

    i.   Provide ventilations.

    ii. Reassess every 30 seconds.

3. Heart rate above 100: Assess skin color.

H. Assess skin color. If central cyanosis is present, provide blow-by oxygen at about 4 to 6 lpm with oxygen tubing near the baby's face until color improves.

I. APGAR Score

1. Attempt to obtain APGAR score at one minute and five minutes after delivery of the baby.

2. **A**ppearance

    i.   0 points: cyanotic all over

    ii. 1 point: core pink, but hands and feet cyanotic

    iii. 2 points: pink all over

3. **P**ulse

    i.   0 points: no pulse

    ii. 1 point: heart rate under 100

    iii. 2 points: heart rate over 100

4. **G**rimace (stimulation reflex)

    i.   0 points: no response to stimulation

    ii. 1 point: minimal (facial grimace) response to stimulation

    iii. 2 points: responds vigorously, such as crying

5. **A**ctivity (extremity movement)

    i.   0 points: limp

    ii. 1 point: limited active movement

    iii. 2 points: actively moving

6. **R**espirations

    i.   0 points: not breathing

    ii. 1 point: slow or irregular breathing

    iii. 2 points: adequate breathing

VIII. DELIVERY COMPLICATIONS

A. Meconium

1. Meconium is the presence of fetal stool in the amniotic fluid. This turns the amniotic fluid yellow, green, or brownish.

2. The risk of infection and pneumonia increases if the baby inhales meconium.

3. If meconium is present, suction the mouth and nose promptly when the head clears the birth canal.

4. Once the baby delivers, immediately suction the mouth and nose prior to stimulating the baby to breathe.

B. Multiple Births

1. Multiple births can have their own placenta, or share a placenta.

2. Be prepared for multiple births any time it has not been ruled out by ultrasound.

3. Request additional units.

4. Prepare additional supplies, OB kits, bag valve masks (BVMs), oxygen tanks, etc.

5. Be prepared for possible breech presentation, particularly with second baby.

6. Multiple-birth babies may be smaller and require additional resuscitation efforts.

7. Clamp and cut an umbilical cord with possible multiple births only as a last resort.

8. If second baby does not deliver within about 10 minutes after first, transport immediately.

C. Prolapsed Cord

1. A prolapsed cord occurs when the cord is the presenting part in the birth canal.

2. A prolapsed cord can become compressed and cut off oxygen to the baby.

3. Instruct the mother not to push. This will increase pressure on the cord.

4. Place mother in knee-chest position.

5. Carefully push the presenting part of the baby away from the cord.

6. Transport immediately.

D. Breech Presentation

1. A breech birth occurs when the baby's buttocks or legs are the first presenting part in the birth canal.

2. Transport immediately. Breech births present significant dangers for mother and baby.

3. If delivery occurs, there is a high risk the head will become stuck in the birth canal.

4. If the head is trapped, use fingers to form a "V" along vaginal wall to create space allowing the baby to breath.

E. Limb Presentation

1. A limb presentation is when a single arm or leg is the first presenting part in the birth canal.

2. Do *not* attempt delivery of a limb presentation in the field.

3. Place the mother in the knee-chest position and transport immediately.

F. Postpartum Hemorrhage

1. Postpartum hemorrhage is excessive bleeding following delivery.

2. Blood loss of greater than about 500 mL is considered abnormal.

3. Management of postpartum hemorrhage includes uterine massage, breastfeeding, and treating for shock.

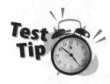

Test Tip

Be sure you know the three key assessments for newborns: respirations, heart rate, and color. Getting the newborn's heart rate above 100 beats per minute and keeping it there is essential.

PRACTICE QUESTIONS

1. Which of the following statements regarding cardiovascular changes in the pregnant patient is correct?

   A. During pregnancy, the cardiac workload decreases.

   B. Pregnant patients are at an increased risk of anemia.

   C. Signs of shock are more obvious in the pregnant patient.

   D. Postural hypotension is uncommon in pregnant patients.

2. Which of the following is a common cause of bleeding in the pregnant patient during the third trimester?

   A. placenta previa

   B. preeclampsia

   C. pregnancy-induced hypertension

   D. supine hypotensive syndrome

3. Your patient is 37 weeks pregnant. She is complaining of headache, blurred vision, and swelling. You should suspect

   A. preeclampsia.

   B. eclampsia.

   C. ectopic pregnancy.

   D. uterine rupture.

4. Your pregnant patient states her blood pressure has been high each of the last three times she has checked it. You should suspect

   A. supine hypotensive syndrome.

   B. eclampsia.

   C. pregnancy-induced hypertension.

   D. ectopic pregnancy.

5. Your patient is 37 weeks pregnant. You find her supine in bed complaining of weakness and nausea. You should immediately be concerned about

A. a hypertensive crisis.

B. gestational diabetes.

C. domestic abuse.

D. supine hypotensive syndrome.

ANSWERS

1. **B.**

   RBC production increases in pregnant patients, but plasma increase is greater. This leads to a relative anemia.

2. **A.**

   Placenta previa is a common cause of vaginal bleeding during the third trimester of pregnancy.

3. **A.**

   Preeclampsia occurs in the third trimester and presents with sudden weight gain, visual disturbances, sudden swelling of the face, hands, or feet, headache, and hypertension.

4. **C.**

   PIH is defined as a blood pressure in a pregnant patient above 140/90 at least twice over several hours.

5. **D.**

   Patients in the later stages of pregnancy should NOT be positioned supine due to the risk of supine hypotensive syndrome.

Pediatric Emergencies

I. ANATOMY AND PHYSIOLOGY OF PEDIATRICS

A. Airway/Respiratory

1. Tongue. Infants have a proportionally larger tongue than adults. This allows little room for swelling.

2. Lower airway. The pediatric lower airway is smaller and more easily obstructed.

3. Obligate nose breathers. Most newborns and infants breathe through their nose, not mouth. Respiratory distress can develop rapidly if the nares are obstructed.

B. Head

1. The pediatric patient's head is proportionally larger in relation to the body than an adult's head.

2. The head is a significant source of heat loss.

3. Pediatric patients are at an increased risk of head trauma.

4. Padding is typically required behind the shoulders to immobilize a pediatric patient in a neutral, in-line position.

5. A sunken fontanelle in infants may indicate hypovolemia. A bulging fontanelle may indicate increased intracranial pressure.

6. Children require a greater cerebral blood flow. Hypoxia can develop rapidly.

C. Chest

1. Ribs are more pliable in pediatric patients, decreasing risk of rib fractures and increasing risk of internal injury.

2. Smaller lungs require lower tidal volumes during artificial ventilation. There is an increased risk of injury due to overinflation.

3. Pediatrics are often abdominal breathers.

D. Abdomen. Organs are less protected and more anterior. This makes a pediatric patient more susceptible to injury.

E. Cardiovascular

1. Bradycardia should be regarded as a sign of hypoxia in the pediatric patient.

2. Hypotension does not typically develop until the pediatric patient is significantly hypovolemic and then crashes rapidly.

F. Metabolic. Pediatric patients typically use oxygen and glucose faster than adults do.

G. Skin

1. The pediatric patient's skin surface is larger in comparison to body mass than an adult's.

2. Pediatrics are more susceptible to hypothermia.

3. Pediatrics have their own Rule of Nines for calculating total body surface areas (TBSA). (See chapter 24.)

II. PEDIATRIC ASSESSMENT TRIANGLE (PAT): THE KEY ASSESSMENTS

A. Appearance (TICLS)

1. Abnormal findings here indicate a possible neurological problem.

2. Assess for TICLS.

   i. Tone. Assess for movement, muscle tone, listlessness, etc.

   ii. Interactivity. Assess for alertness, reactivity to stimulus, interaction with the environment.

   iii. Consolability. Can the child be consoled by the parents or caregivers?

   iv. Look. Is child able to fix his/her gaze, or do they appear "out of it"?

  v. **S**peech or cry. Assess speech in older children, strength of cry in younger patients.

 B. Work of Breathing

  1. Abnormal findings here indicate a respiratory problem.

  2. Assess how hard the child is working to breathe; look for signs and symptoms such as accessory muscle use, abnormal lung sounds, grunting, tripod positional breathing, head bobbing, and nasal flaring.

 C. Circulation to Skin

  1. Abnormal findings here indicate a possible cardiac problem or shock.

  2. Assess skin color: pale, cyanotic, mottled, flushed, jaundice.

 D. Key Points About the PAT

  1. The PAT is intended to be a quick, visual assessment to help determine which pediatric patients require rapid intervention and transport.

  2. You should be able to complete the three key assessments and identify high priority patients in about 30 seconds.

 III. **SUDDEN INFANT DEATH SYNDROME (SIDS)**

 A. SIDS is an unexplained, unexpected death of a patient under one year of age.

 B. SIDS applies only to deaths that cannot be otherwise explained by autopsy.

 C. Prehospital providers do *not* diagnose SIDS. Treat as any other infant cardiac arrest patient and provide emotional support for the family.

 IV. **CHILD ABUSE**

 A. Physical abuse is excessive or inappropriate physical force.

 B. Neglect is failure to provide adequate attention when responsible for doing so.

C. Signs of abuse or neglect include obvious trauma, injuries in various stages of healing, unexplained injuries, injuries that do not appear to match the description of how they occurred, and signs of malnutrition.

D. Shaken baby syndrome is a form of abuse caused by violent shaking of a pediatric patient.

E. Management of Suspected Child Abuse

1. Do your best to gain access to the child with the care provider's consent.

2. Examine child as thoroughly as possible.

3. Do not confront the child about what happened in front of possible abusers.

4. Do your best to obtain consent to transport the child to the hospital.

5. Do *not* confront those you suspect of abuse.

6. Request assistance from law enforcement if needed.

7. Report suspected abuse to the appropriate authorities.

8. Document findings objectively.

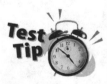
Test Tip

A great deal of information about pediatric patients has been provided in the previous chapters. This chapter enriches the information previously provided; it does not repeat it. Make sure you review the previous chapters for information related to pediatric patients, and update your flashcards accordingly.

Be sure you know the Pediatric Assessment Triangle (PAT). Remember, 15% of the questions on the national certification exam will relate to pediatric patients.

PRACTICE QUESTIONS

1. You are assessing a pediatric patient with bradycardia and an altered LOC. Your immediate priority should be

   A. a complete and thorough secondary assessment.

   B. assessment and management of suspected hypoxia.

   C. placement of the AED on the patient for further analysis.

   D. administration of oral glucose for suspected hypoglycemia.

2. Which of the following is one of the three key assessments of the Pediatric Assessment Triangle?

   A. airway

   B. baseline vitals

   C. appearance

   D. control bleeding

3. Which of the following statements is correct regarding management of a pediatric patient you suspect has been abused?

   A. You are legally required to report suspected abuse to the appropriate authorities.

   B. You can only report suspected abuse to your direct supervisor.

   C. You are not permitted to report suspected abuse without a guardian's consent.

   D. You must have proof of physical abuse before reporting your suspicions.

4. Select the correct statement regarding the Rule of Nines for pediatric patients.

   A. The Rule of Nines for pediatric patients is the same as for adults.

   B. The pediatric Rule of Nines assigns a higher percentage to the legs.

   C. The pediatric Rule of Nines assigns a higher percentage to the head.

   D. The Rule of Nines should not be applied to pediatric patients under 10 years of age.

5. Which of the following statements regarding SIDS is correct?

    A. SIDS is any non traumatic cardiac arrest in pediatric patients.

    B. SIDS only occurs in patients over 1 year of age.

    C. SIDS is easily identifiable upon autopsy.

    D. SIDS only applies to deaths that cannot be explained by autopsy.

ANSWERS

1. **B.**

    Bradycardia should be regarded as a sign of hypoxia in pediatric patients. The AED should not be applied to a patient that is not in cardiac arrest. Administration of oral glucose should take place after management of hypoxia and determination of the patient's blood glucose level when possible.

2. **C.**

    The three key assessments of the PAT are appearance, work of breathing, and circulation to skin.

3. **A.**

    EMS providers are legally required to report suspected abuse to the appropriate authorities.

4. **C.**

    The pediatric Rule of Nines assigns a higher percentage to the head and a lower percentage to the legs compared to the adult Rule of Nines.

5. **D.**

    SIDS is an unexplained, unexpected death of a patient under one year of age. SIDS applies only to deaths that cannot be otherwise explained by autopsy.

Geriatric Patients

I. CONSIDERATIONS FOR THE GERIATRIC PATIENT POPULATION

A. Communication

1. Speak clearly, and ask only one question at a time.

2. Do not assume the patient is hard of hearing or doesn't understand what you are saying. Speak *to* them, not *about* them.

3. Be patient. Geriatric patients often understand you, but need additional time to respond.

B. Medical History

1. Hypertension, heart disease, and diabetes are just a few of the medical conditions common to geriatric patients.

2. The patient's current health, medical history, and medications can cause conditions that wouldn't be as serious in younger patients to present significant risks to the geriatric patient.

C. Medications

1. Geriatric patients are often on multiple medications (polypharmacy), sometimes from different physicians. These medications can have dangerous interactions.

2. Medications can easily be mismanaged by geriatric patients if they are unsure how to take them, forget to take them, accidentally overdose on them, or simply can't afford them.

D. Mechanism of Injury (MOI)

1. Physiological changes in geriatric patients increase the risk of injury due to trauma.

        i.   An MOI that may be of lesser concern in a younger patient can be life threatening to a geriatric patient.

        ii. Your index of suspicion for geriatric patients should be much higher. The MOI needed to cause significant trauma is much lower. Even ground-level falls can be extremely dangerous.

  2. Taking spinal precautions can be challenging. Some geriatric patients are unable to lie flat due to spinal abnormalities such as kyphosis (a curvature of the spine that leads to a rounded back).

  3. Always investigate the cause of trauma with a geriatric patient. There may be a more serious medical condition that led to the injury (for example, palpitations or syncope leading to a fall injury).

E. Environmental Cues

  1. Understand that you are one of the few health care providers that will see the patient's living conditions. This provides a great deal of information.

  2. Does the patient reside in a safe environment?

  3. Are their signs of neglect, abuse, malnutrition?

  4. Does the patient live alone?

  5. Does the patient appear to be equipped to handle the tasks of daily living?

  6. Leading causes of death include heart disease, stroke, cancer, and trauma.

II. SPECIFIC MEDICAL CONDITIONS

A. Myocardial Infarction (MI)

  1. Maintain high index of suspicion for cardiac problems in geriatric patients.

  2. Geriatric patients frequently present with atypical (unusual) signs and symptoms when experiencing an MI.

  3. Geriatric patients may complain of weakness, dyspnea, abdominal pain, or epigastric pain instead of chest pain.

  4. "Silent MIs" (no complaint of chest pain) are more common in the geriatric population, especially diabetics and females.

B. Congestive Heart Failure (CHF)

   1. Geriatric patients are at higher risk for CHF, especially those with hypertension, previous MIs, and coronary artery disease.

   2. Left-sided heart failure

      i. Left heart failure causes fluid to back up into the lungs.

      ii. Left heart failure typically presents with pulmonary edema and respiratory distress.

   3. Right-sided heart failure

      i. Right heart failure causes fluid to back up into the body.

      ii. Right heart failure typically presents with pedal edema and jugular venous distention (JVD).

   4. CHF patients frequently complain of weakness, dyspnea (especially upon exertion), and difficulty breathing at night while lying down.

C. Pneumonia

   1. Pneumonia is a potentially life-threatening infection in the lungs.

   2. Geriatric patients are at higher risk for pneumonia, especially those that are chronically ill.

   3. General weakness, fever, cough, and dyspnea are common complaints of those experiencing pneumonia.

D. Pulmonary Embolism (PE)

   1. PE is caused by a blockage of a pulmonary artery. This compromises blood flow to the lungs.

   2. Common signs and symptoms include fatigue, chest pain, tachycardia, sudden onset dyspnea, pedal edema in only one leg, low pulse oximetry readings, and a general feeling of distress.

   3. In some cases, the presentation may be subtle; however, PE can lead to sudden cardiac arrest.

   4. Risk factors include long sedentary periods (such as a long-distance flight), recent surgery, or long-bone fractures, a history of blood clots, and obesity.

   5. High-flow oxygen should be provided to patients with a suspected PE.

E. Deep Vein Thrombosis (DVT)

    1. DVT is a blood clot in a large vein, usually in the leg.

    2. A loose clot (embolus) can cause a pulmonary embolism.

    3. Long-term immobility (such as travel, hospitalization, sedentary lifestyle) can increase the risk of DVT and PE.

F. Cerebrovascular Accident (CVA; Stroke)

    1. Stroke is common in the geriatric population.

    2. A stroke assessment (such as Cincinnati Stroke Scale) should be performed on any patient with a suspected CVA. Suspected stroke patients are a high-priority transport and should be taken to an appropriate facility for rapid intervention. (See chapter 16 for additional information.)

G. GI Disorders

    1. Geriatric patients are at an increased risk for GI bleeds and aortic aneurysm.

    2. Maintain a high index of suspicion for any geriatric patient with abdominal pain.

    3. Assess for vomiting blood; coffee-ground-like emesis; bloody stool; dark, tarry stool; severe back or flank pain; pulsating abdominal mass; and signs and symptoms of shock.

H. Dementia

    1. Dementia is a slow, progressive deterioration on cognitive function.

    2. Stroke, Alzheimer's disease, and various genetic disorders can lead to dementia.

    3. Dementia patients often present with hallucinations, aggressive behavior, a limited attention span, diminished motor or social skills, and reduced cognitive abilities.

I. Delirium

    1. Unlike dementia, delirium is a sudden change in cognitive function or mental status.

    2. Unlike dementia, delirium can often be treated and reversed.

3. Delirium patients may experience acute anxiety; however, their memory is often unaffected.

J. Depression

1. Depression and suicide rates are high among geriatric patients.

2. Depression is especially high among geriatric patients living in nursing facilities.

3. Geriatric females have higher rates of depression; however, males have higher suicide rates.

4. Geriatric patients who attempt suicide are more likely to be successful than younger adults.

5. Suicide risk factors include chronic illness or pain, terminal illness, death of a spouse, and loss of independence.

K. Trauma

1. The risk of death from all forms of trauma is greater in the geriatric population.

2. Pelvic and femur fractures are extremely dangerous in the geriatric population. The risk of shock, pneumonia, and pulmonary embolism is high following a pelvic or femur fracture.

3. Be alert for signs of elderly neglect or abuse.

L. Osteoporosis

1. Osteoporosis is the progressive loss of bone density over time.

2. It is more common in females and often leads to hip and other fractures.

3. A calcium deficiency often leads to osteoporosis.

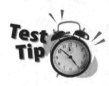
Test Tip

For many of the questions on the certification exam, you will likely think there are two possible correct answers. With careful consideration, you should be able to identify one of the four as the best choice. Start by rereading the question and each answer choice carefully. Keep in mind that you're not looking for the perfect answer. You are looking for the best choice among those provided.

When you think there are two correct answers, reread the question. It will almost always give you a clue as to which is the better choice.

PRACTICE QUESTIONS

1. Your elderly patient has a curvature of the spine that causes her to have a rounded back. This is known as

    A. spondylosis.

    B. kyphosis.

    C. lordosis.

    D. scoliosis.

2. Your elderly female patient complains of weakness and non-specific abdominal pain. You should maintain a high index of suspicion for

    A. gastroenteritis.

    B. food poisoning.

    C. atypical MI.

    D. diverticulitis.

3. Your elderly patient presents with pulmonary edema and respiratory distress. The patient has a history of hypertension and two previous MIs. You should suspect

    A. left heart failure.

    B. right heart failure.

    C. COPD.

    D. pulmonary embolism.

4. Your elderly patient is overweight and recently had surgery for a long-bone fracture. He has decided to take a 12-hour flight overseas to relax and recover. This patient has multiple risk factors for

    A. cardiac tamponade.

    B. chronic obstructive pulmonary disease.

    C. pulmonary embolism.

    D. status asthmaticus.

5. Your elderly patient complains of abdominal pain, coffee-ground-like emesis, and dark, tarry stool. You should suspect

   A. ingestion of coffee grounds.

   B. a stomach flu.

   C. a bowel obstruction.

   D. GI bleeding.

ANSWERS

1. **B.**

   Kyphosis is a curvature of the spine that leads to a rounded back. Lordosis and scoliosis are also abnormal curvatures of the spine. Spondylosis is age-related wear to the spinal disks.

2. **C.**

   Geriatric patients often present with atypical symptoms of MI, especially females.

3. **A.**

   Pulmonary edema and dyspnea are indications of left heart failure. HTN and previous MIs are risk factors for CHF. Pulmonary edema is more common with CHF than COPD or pulmonary embolism.

4. **C.**

   Risk factors for pulmonary embolism include long sedentary periods (such as a long-distance flight), recent surgery, long-bone fractures, a history of blood clots, and obesity.

5. **D.**

   Signs and symptoms of GI bleeding include vomiting blood, coffee-ground-like emesis, bloody stool, dark, tarry stool, severe back or flank pain, pulsating abdominal mass, and signs and symptoms of shock.

Special Patient Populations

33

I. SPECIAL CHALLENGES

A. Patients with special challenges, as well as their families, may need emotional support as well as medical attention.

B. Hearing Impaired

1. Face the patient and speak clearly.

2. Consider communicating in writing.

3. A family member may be able to assist.

4. Consider use of more closed-ended questions.

C. Vision Impaired

1. Communicate verbally what you are doing.

2. Keep the patient informed about what is going on around them.

3. Protect the patient from harm when moving them.

D. Speech Impaired

1. Ask questions that allow concise answers.

2. Do not attempt to finish the patient's statements for them.

3. Allow patient additional time to respond to questions.

4. Do not pretend you understand what they are saying if you do not.

E. Developmental Disabilities

1. There are many causes of developmental disabilities, but most affect the central nervous system in some way.

2. Do not assume that the patient's appearance is an indication of their cognitive function.

3. Attempt to communicate with the patient and keep them informed.

4. The patient's family or care provider may be a valuable resource. Keep them nearby.

5. Attempt to determine how the patient's current presentation differs from their baseline.

F. Brain-Injured Patients

1. These patients often rely on extensive medical equipment, such as ventilators, infusion pumps, feeding tubes, and catheters.

2. Use caution when manipulating medical equipment. If unsure, consult care providers if present, ALS providers, or medical direction.

3. Airway and respiratory problems, such as obstruction and pneumonia, are common.

4. Bed sores, urinary tract infections, and malnutrition are common problems.

G. Dialysis Patients

1. Dialysis patients require mechanical assistance to filter their blood supply due to poor kidney function.

2. Dialysis patients typically have an implanted device, such as an arteriovenous (AV) shunt, fistula, or graft. Do *not* take a blood pressure on an extremity with such a device.

3. Monitor dialysis patients closely for signs of shock or infection.

H. Obesity

1. Obese patients can present challenges related to assessment, management, and transport.

2. Many EMS systems have specialized bariatric ambulances to assist with movement and transport of obese patients.

3. Some equipment may not be sized adequately for the patient.

4. Airway management, ventilations, chest compressions, and cervical-spine (c-spine) stabilization can be especially challenging.

I. Terminally Ill Patients

    1. Terminally ill patients have a disease that is likely to get progressively worse until death.

    2. Hospice facilities are specialty facilities designed to provide comfort care to terminally ill patients.

    3. Make every effort to comfort terminally ill patients and their family.

II. SPECIAL EQUIPMENT

A. Tracheostomy

    1. A tracheostomy is a surgical procedure that creates an opening through the neck into the trachea.

    2. A stoma is a surgical opening into the trachea.

    3. A tracheostomy tube can be placed in the stoma and connects to a ventilator or bag valve mask (BVM). Tracheostomy tubes can become obstructed easily by secretions. Be prepared to suction with a French suction catheter.

    4. Patients with a tracheostomy ventilate through their stoma, not the mouth or nose.

    5. Supplemental oxygen should be applied over the stoma using a tracheostomy mask (not common in the prehospital environment) or a nonrebreather mask.

B. Home Ventilators

    1. Home ventilators may allow control of rate, tidal volume, and oxygen concentration.

    2. Do not manipulate ventilator settings without proper training and medical direction authorization.

    3. Family or home care providers are often familiar with the patient's equipment and its operation.

    4. If you suspect a ventilator malfunction, immediately begin ventilations with a BVM.

C. Analgesia Pump

    1. A patient-controlled analgesia (PCA) pump is a device that allows patients to self-administer pain medication through infusion.

2. The pain medication is typically locked within the device, and there is a limit to how much medication the patient can self-administer at one time.

3. Some EMS systems allow EMTs to monitor and transport a patient with an analgesia pump. Consult local protocol and medical direction.

D. Apnea Monitor

1. An apnea monitor is a device that continuously monitors a patient's breathing and alarms if breathing stops for a period of time.

2. If the patient is on an apnea monitor, determine if it went off, when, and how often.

3. Determine if any interventions (ventilations, CPR) were provided prior to your arrival.

E. Vascular Access Device (VAD)

1. A VAD is used for patients who require ongoing venous access for mediations, dialysis, chemotherapy, etc.

2. EMTs do not use VADs as a route for medications.

3. Do *not* take a blood pressure on an extremity with a VAD.

F. Feeding Tubes

1. Feeding tubes go from the nose (nasogastric) or mouth (orogastric) into the stomach and provide a route for nutrition when patients can't chew or swallow.

2. Nasogastric (NG) and orogastric (OG) tubes can also be used to remove air or toxins from the stomach.

G. Colostomy. Patients with various gastrointestinal (GI) problems may have a surgical opening in their abdominal wall that allows feces to exit without traveling through the entire GI tract and out the colon.

H. Foley Catheter

1. A foley catheter is placed into the urethra and allows urine to drain into a bag.

2. The patient is at risk for infection without proper hygiene.

3. Use extreme caution when moving a patient with a foley catheter. Keep the catheter positioned low to allow drainage into the collection bag.

I. Intraventricular Shunt

1. An intraventricular shunt allows excess cerebrospinal fluid (CSF) to exit the ventricles of the brain.

2. Intraventricular shunts can become obstructed and allow a dangerous increase in intracranial pressure. There is also the risk of infection and bleeding.

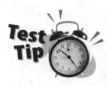
Test Tip

The latest National EMS Practice Analysis can be purchased through the NREMT. The practice analysis provides information about the most important EMS-related tasks and the current standards for appropriate patient care. For additional information about the National EMS Practice Analysis, visit www.nremt.org.

PRACTICE QUESTIONS

1. Your patient receives dialysis and has an AV shunt on the left arm. You should

   A. take all blood pressures on the left arm.

   B. avoid taking blood pressures on the left arm.

   C. delay taking any blood pressures until ALS arrives.

   D. ask the patient which arm should be used for blood pressures.

2. Your patient has a tracheostomy tube and presents with signs of hypoxia. You suspect the tube is partially obstructed. You should

   A. remove the tracheostomy tube.

   B. place the patient on a nasal cannula.

   C. perform abdominal thrusts.

   D. suction the tracheostomy tube.

3. Your patient has a stoma and requires supplemental oxygen. You should

   A. contact medical direction before administering supplemental oxygen.

   B. apply a nasal cannula set to a maximum of 6 lpm.

   C. place an oxygen mask over the stoma.

   D. administer oxygen via NRB as normal.

4. Your patient is on a home ventilator. The ventilator appears to be malfunctioning. You should immediately

   A. begin ventilating the patient with a BVM.

   B. contact medical control for instructions.

   C. try resetting the power on the ventilator.

   D. increase the tidal volume on the ventilator.

5. Your hospice patient has a PCA pump. The PCA pump is used to

   A. self-administer pain medication.

   B. administer medications intravenously.

   C. facilitate renal dialysis.

   D. improve cardiac output.

ANSWERS

1. **B.**

   Do NOT take blood pressures on an arm with an AV shunt, fistula, or graft.

2. **D.**

   Tracheostomy tubes often become obstructed by secretions.

3. **C.**

   Supplemental oxygen should be applied over the stoma using a mask.

4. **A.**

   If you suspect a ventilator malfunction, immediately begin ventilations with a BVM.

5. **A.**

   A patient-controlled analgesia pump is a device that allows the patient to self-administer pain medication.

PART VII

EMS
OPERATIONS

Ambulance and Air Medical Operations

I. AMBULANCE DESIGN

A. Contemporary ambulances should meet all of the following criteria:

1. Separate compartments for driver and patient

2. Room for at least two EMS providers and two patients

3. All necessary medical equipment for the scope of practice being provided

4. Radio communication with dispatchers, and the capability to establish online medical direction

5. Compliant with local and federal safety requirements

6. Compliant with local ambulance certification requirements

7. Typically, a displayed six-pointed "Star of Life" emblem

B. Ambulance Types

1. Type I ambulance: truck chassis with modular ambulance body

2. Type II ambulance: standard van design

3. Type III ambulance: specialty van design with a square patient compartment mounted on the chassis

II. PHASES OF AN AMBULANCE CALL

A. Preparation Phase. Inspect the ambulance every day and after each shift change.

B. Dispatch. Determine the nature of the call, location, and number of patients.

C. En Route to Scene

1. Notify dispatch you are responding.

2. Operate the ambulance according to state and local laws and agency policies.

3. *All* emergency vehicle operators must drive with due regard for the safety of others.

D. Arrival at Scene/Patient Contact

1. Notify dispatch you are on scene.

2. Upon arrival at a scene, the ambulance should be positioned to allow for safe egress and patient loading.

3. If necessary, use the ambulance as a barrier to protect the scene.

4. The ambulance may be used to provide additional lighting if needed.

E. Patient Transfer to Ambulance. The patient must be properly secured for transport.

F. Transport to Receiving Facility

1. Notify dispatch you are transporting the patient and specify where.

2. Notify the receiving hospital according to local protocol.

3. Determine whether emergency transport is warranted.

4. Confirm patient is being transported to appropriate receiving facility.

G. Arrival at Hospital/Transfer of Care

1. Notify dispatch you have arrived at the hospital.

2. Provide verbal report to appropriate hospital personnel of equal or higher medical authority.

3. Provide copy of written patient care record.

4. Obtain signature verifying transfer of care.

H. Postrun Phase/Return to Service

　　1. Ensure all necessary equipment is restocked and ready for use on the next call.

　　2. Ensure ambulance and equipment is adequately cleaned, disinfected, or sterilized per local protocol.

III. DEFENSIVE DRIVING TACTICS

A. The quality of patient care is far more important than the speed of the response. Do *not* sacrifice safety for speed.

B. Everyone must be properly restrained whenever the vehicle is traveling.

C. All equipment should be properly secured.

D. Emergency vehicles should usually travel in the far left lane.

E. Always know what is next to you while driving.

F. Scan the road frequently and several car lengths ahead of you.

G. Allow several vehicle lengths distance between you and the vehicle ahead of you, when possible.

H. Anticipate unexpected actions from other motorists.

I. Always assume other drivers do not see or hear you.

J. Pass on the left when possible.

K. Use extreme caution when backing up. Always use a spotter.

L. Remember you have blind spots and minimize them as best you're able.

M. Recognize that ambulances typically have a high center of gravity. Take corners carefully.

N. Be especially cautious while driving in bad weather, poor visibility, and at night.

O. Use daytime running lights according to local protocol.

P. Lights and sirens should be used together.

Q. Recognize fatigue as a significant threat to safe vehicle operation.

IV. AIR AMBULANCE

A. Types of Air Ambulances

1. Air ambulances may include rotor-wing aircraft (helicopters) or fixed-wing aircraft (planes).

2. Fixed-wing aircraft are typically used for longer distances (at least 100 to 150 miles) and require a runway for safe takeoff and landing.

B. Landing Zones for Rotor-Wing Aircraft

1. Takeoff and landing is the most dangerous part of flight.

2. The landing zone (LZ) should be secured well before the rotor-wing aircraft arrives and should remain secured until the aircraft is completely clear of the scene and traveling away.

3. The LZ should measure at least 100 feet by 100 feet and be on firm, level ground.

4. Ensure there are no overhead obstructions near the LZ, such as power lines.

5. Clear all loose debris away from the LZ.

6. There should be radio contact between the aircraft and someone on the ground to relay critical information during approach, landing, and takeoff.

C. Operating Around Rotor-Wing Aircraft

1. Never approach the aircraft without permission or from the rear.

2. Make sure all loose items are secured before approaching a running aircraft or loading patients.

3. Be familiar with local protocols related to air-medical operations. Not all patients can or should be transported by air.

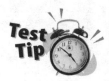

Remember—Safety First! You are likely to see a number of safety-related questions on the certification exam. Pay particular attention to safety information while reviewing the operations chapters.

PRACTICE QUESTIONS

1. Following a call, you clean and disinfect all of the equipment used. This occurs during the

   A. transfer of care phase of a call.

   B. postrun phase of a call.

   C. preparation phase of a call.

   D. transport phase of a call.

2. Emergency vehicles should usually travel

   A. in the far right lane.

   B. in the center lane.

   C. in the far left lane.

   D. in the widest lane.

3. Which of the following is a recommended defensive driving tactic for emergency vehicle operators?

   A. Follow closely behind larger vehicles in order to "draft."

   B. Focus intensively on the vehicle immediately ahead of you.

   C. Always assume other drivers do not hear or see you.

   D. Try to pass on the right whenever possible.

4. You have been asked to set up a landing zone for an incoming EMS helicopter. You should

   A. ensure the LZ is clear of overhead obstructions.

   B. obtain a local weather report and relay it to the pilot.

   C. place a strobe in the center of the LZ.

   D. select an LZ that is 50 feet by 50 feet.

5. When working around an EMS helicopter, you should NEVER approach the aircraft

   A. while it is running.

   B. from the nose.

   C. until the engine starts.

   D. from the rear.

ANSWERS

1. **B.**

   During the postrun or return to service phase, you restock equipment and clean and disinfect equipment used.

2. **C.**

   Emergency vehicles should usually travel in the far left lane in the event an emergency response is required.

3. **C.**

   You should always assume other drivers do not hear or see you and anticipate unexpected actions.

4. **A.**

   The LZ should be at least 100 feet by 100 feet and clear of obstructions. A strobe in the center of the LZ may obstruct the pilot's vision and create a landing hazard.

5. **D.**

   Never approach the aircraft from the rear because the pilot can't see you and the tail rotor is an extreme hazard.

Vehicle Extrication

I. SAFETY DURING VEHICLE EXTRICATION OPERATIONS

A. The EMT's primary responsibilities at a scene involving vehicle extrication or special operations are personal safety and delivery of patient care once it is safe to do so.

B. Do not attempt extrication procedures you have not been trained for or are not equipped to handle.

C. As always, gloves and eye protection are required.

D. Leather gloves should also be used over (not instead of) regular gloves if handling glass, sharp objects, rope, etc.

E. Federal law requires EMS workers wear an approved highly reflective traffic safety vest when working on roadways, around traffic, or at an accident scene.

II. VEHICLE SAFETY SYSTEMS

A. Shock-Absorbing Bumpers

   1. Most vehicles today are equipped with shock-absorbing bumpers (front and rear).

   2. They can become compressed during an accident and spontaneously release, injuring anyone standing in front of them.

   3. Approach vehicles from the sides, not the front.

   4. Do *not* conduct patient care in front of or behind vehicles.

B. Supplemental Restraint System (SRS)

1. Most vehicles today are equipped with SRS airbags.

2. Airbags inflate at up to 200 miles per hour if triggered during an accident.

3. Front airbags typically begin deflating as soon as they are fully inflated. Side-impact airbags may remain inflated longer due to the possibility of a rollover.

4. Airbags not previously deployed may inflate spontaneously after an accident. This poses a risk to anyone within the vehicle, such as EMTs caring for patients.

5. Maintain about two feet of clearance between you and undeployed airbags whenever possible.

6. Assume airbags can still deploy even after the car battery has been disconnected.

7. Children under 12 years of age should *not* be placed in the front seat of a vehicle with SRS airbags.

8. *Never* place an infant in the front seat of a vehicle with an SRS airbag.

9. Occupants may experience minor abrasions or contusions due to airbag deployment. Orthopedic injury to the hands or arms of drivers may also occur due to airbag deployment.

10. When assessing the mechanism of injury (MOI), remember to look under deployed airbags when it is safe to do so.

III. PHASES OF EXTRICATION

A. Preparation. Ensure appropriate training, equipment, etc.

B. En Route to Scene

C. Arrival

1. Position vehicle in a safe location. Use vehicle to increase scene safety if needed.

2. Assess the scene for hazards, number of patients, etc.

3. Perform a 360-degree walk-around if safe to do so.

D. Control of Hazards

    1. Examples include traffic, downed power lines, fuel leaks, and hazardous materials.

    2. It is common practice to disconnect the vehicle's battery during extrication operations. Do not attempt this without proper training. Electric vehicles and alternative-fuel vehicles can present special challenges and hazards.

E. Support Ops. Examples include scene lighting, helicopter landing zones, and staging areas.

F. Gaining Access

    1. EMTs without additional training do not typically gain access to patients if there are special hazards, specialized tools, or equipment required.

    2. EMTs may assist in keeping the patient safe while rescuers attempt to gain access or extricate the patient. This may include providing eye protection or covering with a blanket.

G. Patient Care

    1. If safe to do so, patient care may begin before extrication is completed.

    2. Perform a standard primary assessment by taking manual cervical-spine (c-spine) precautions and assessing airway, breathing, and circulation (ABCs).

H. Removal of Patient

    1. Simple access: gaining access to the patient without any tools or the need to break glass.

    2. Complex access

        i. Complex access requires the use of special tools and training.

        ii. EMTs without additional training should not attempt complex access.

    3. Extrication: the removal of the patient from entrapment.

    4. Entrapment: when a person is trapped in an enclosed space.

5. Removing a patient from a damaged vehicle, especially with c-spine precautions, can be challenging and labor intensive. Several rescuers are often required.

6. Emergency move: used when the scene is dangerous and the patient must be moved immediately and before providing patient care.

7. Urgent move

   i.   Used when the patient has potentially life-threatening injuries or illness and must be moved quickly for evaluation and transport.

   ii. Rapid extrication

        ➤ An urgent move used for patients in a motor vehicle.

        ➤ Requires multiple rescuers and a long backboard.

        ➤ Patient is rotated onto a long spine board with manual c-spine and removed from vehicle.

I. Patient Transfer. Once the patient is freed, perform a complete assessment.

J. Conclusion of Extrication. Units return to service.

 IV. SPECIAL SITUATIONS

A. Certain situations may present unusual hazards and require specialized personnel. If dispatched to a special rescue situation, stage in a safe location, report to the incident commander upon arrival, and await further instructions.

B. Special rescue situations may include

   1. technical rescue or search and rescue

   2. water rescue

   3. structure fires

   4. tactical situations involving law enforcement operations

   5. hazardous materials incidents

   6. mass casualty incidents

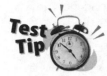

Recent exam results indicate that EMS Operations is one of the most difficult topic areas for many candidates taking the NREMT exam. Consider the following as you decide what priority EMS Operations will have in your study plan:

1. *On the exam, you will likely see fewer questions related to EMS Operations than to the other categories.*

2. *Practices related to many EMS Operations topics vary greatly from one EMS system to the next. Developing test questions that apply to all EMS systems across the country is difficult. However, one of the few consistencies among the various EMS systems is the need to ensure personal safety.*

PRACTICE QUESTIONS

1. What is the EMT's primary responsibility at a scene involving extrication or special operations?

   A. personal safety

   B. establishing a treatment sector

   C. assisting with extrication as directed

   D. assuming incident command

2. When working on roadways or around traffic, federal law requires that you

   A. stop traffic in all directions near the incident.

   B. wear a turnout coat, bunker pants, and helmet.

   C. wear an approved, highly reflective safety vest.

   D. document the location and condition of all vehicles involved.

3. Due to shock-absorbing bumpers, you should approach vehicles involved in an accident from

   A. the front.

   B. the rear.

   C. the sides.

   D. a crouched position.

4. You are caring for a patient involved in a motor vehicle accident. There is an undeployed airbag in the vehicle. You should

    A. tell the patient you cannot assist him until the fire department arrives.

    B. immediately remove the vehicle's battery.

    C. leave the vehicle running at idle.

    D. maintain about 2 feet of clearance between you and the airbag.

5. Gaining access to the patient at an accident scene without any tools or breaking glass is known as

    A. simple access.

    B. complex access.

    C. rapid extrication.

    D. delayed extrication.

ANSWERS

1. **A.**

    The EMT's primary responsibility is personal safety.

2. **C.**

    Federal laws requires workers to wear an approved, highly reflective traffic safety vest when working on roadways, around traffic, or at an accident scene.

3. **C.**

    Approach vehicles from the sides due to the risk of a compressed bumper releasing spontaneously.

4. **D.**

    Maintain about 2 feet of clearance between you and the undeployed airbag when possible. All other answer choices are inappropriate.

5. **A.**

    Gaining access to the patient without tools or the need to break glass is simple access. Complex access requires the use of special tools and training.

Hazardous Materials

I. INTRODUCTION TO HAZARDOUS MATERIALS

A. Hazardous materials (also called hazmats) are solids, liquids, or gases that pose a threat to people, property, or the environment.

B. Risks of exposure to hazardous materials depend on the dose, concentration, route of exposure, and duration of contact.

C. The EMT's primary responsibilities at a hazardous materials incident are personal safety, notification of appropriate authorities, and the safety of the patient and public.

D. Utilize all your senses to stay alert for hazards. If you are close enough to see it, smell it, hear it, taste it, or touch it, you may already be in danger!

II. HAZARDOUS MATERIALS PLACARDS

A. Vehicles containing certain hazardous materials in certain quantities are required to display identification placards.

B. Drivers of vehicles transporting hazardous materials are required to have shipping papers that identify the substance(s) and quantity being transported.

C. Diamond Placards

    1. Placards will typically display a four-digit United Nations (UN) identification number. All UN numbers are listed in the *Emergency Response Guidebook* (ERG), which can be used to identify the substances and access other essential information.

2. Report this information, if possible, when requesting additional resources. Do *not* enter an unsafe area to look for a placard.

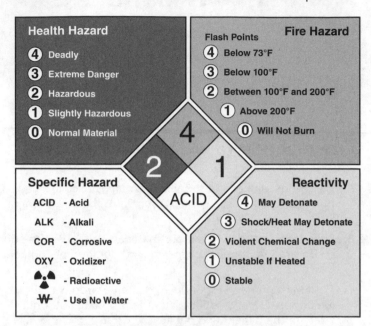

3. Fixed storage locations for hazardous materials should display a diamond placard with four smaller placards within. Each one provides different information through the use of color, numbers, and symbols.

   i.   Blue diamond: provides information about health hazards.

   ii. Red diamond: provides information about fire hazard.

   iii. Yellow diamond: provides information about reactivity hazards.

   iv. White diamond: displays symbols indicating special hazards, such as radioactivity and reactivity to water.

   v.   The higher the number (0 to 4) within the blue, red, or yellow diamonds, the greater the hazard is within that category.

4. Visit the University of Oregon's website (*http://chemlabs.uoregon. edu*) or the National Fire Prevention Association's (NFPA) website (*www.nfpa.org*) for additional information about diamond placards.

III. RESOURCES

A. When in doubt, request additional resources, such as the fire department, law enforcement, and hazardous materials teams.

B. The *Emergency Response Guidebook* can provide essential information.

C. When safe to do so, question the driver and request shipping papers.

D. The Chemical Transportation Emergency Center (CHEMTREC) is available anytime at 1-800-424-9300 in the U.S.

IV. HAZARDOUS MATERIALS TRAINING

A. **First Responder Awareness** trains responders to recognize potential hazards, call for appropriate resources, and prevent others from entering the scene. Federal law requires EMTs receive First Responder Awareness level training.

B. **First Responder Operations** training is designed for those who initially respond to hazmat scenes. Operations-level personnel are trained to protect people, property, and the environment. They are also trained in the use of specialized personal protective equipment (PPE).

C. **Hazardous Materials Technicians** receive significant training related to stopping the release or spread of hazardous materials.

D. **Hazardous Materials Specialists** have the most advanced knowledge and skills. They typically provide assistance at the command level.

V. THE EMT'S TOP TWO PRIORITIES

A. First priority: personal safety

B. Second priority: patient care in a safe zone

VI. SAFE ZONE

A. Hot Zone

1. This is the contaminated area.

2. Appropriate PPE is required, as determined by hazmat personnel.

3. Regardless of patient condition, those without proper training and PPE are *not* permitted in the hot zone.

4. Patient care does not take place in the hot zone.

B. Warm Zone

1. This is the area between the hot and cold zones.

2. Appropriate PPE is required.

3. Only life-threatening conditions are treated in the warm zone.

4. Everyone must be decontaminated in the warm zone before entering the cold zone.

C. Cold Zone

1. Most treatment is performed in the cold zone.

2. Typically, EMS providers remain in the cold zone.

 VII. DECONTAMINATION

A. Decontamination is essential to prevent spreading the hazardous material. Any of the following may become contaminated and require decontamination:

1. The patient's body, hair, clothes, possessions, etc.

2. Medical equipment

3. Emergency vehicle

B. Decontamination should be performed by those properly trained and equipped to do so.

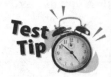

If you are building flashcards in preparation for the NREMT exam, you should be almost done. How soon do you want to take the exam? Divide the number of flashcards you still need to learn by the number of days until you want to test. This will tell you how many flashcards per day you need to learn. Be sure to establish a reasonable timeline for yourself. Try to learn at least five new flashcards every day. Don't forget to regularly review those you already know!

PRACTICE QUESTIONS

1. The UN number on a diamond placard is used to

    A. determine the chemical composition of a hazardous substance.

    B. identify the material's country of origin.

    C. identify the substance using the ERG.

    D. determine the quantity of hazardous materials.

2. A diamond placard with four smaller placards of different colors is used for

    A. fixed storage locations.

    B. commercial transport vehicles.

    C. aircraft with hazardous materials.

    D. cargo ships transporting hazardous materials.

3. The blue diamond on a four-diamond placard provides information about

    A. fire hazards.

    B. special hazards.

    C. reactivity hazards.

    D. health hazards.

4. You see the number 4 within a yellow placard on a four-diamond placard at a storage facility. This means the facility contains

   A. an extreme medical hazard.

   B. normal materials with no known hazards.

   C. a corrosive substance.

   D. a material that may detonate spontaneously.

5. All EMTs are required to have hazardous materials training at the level of

   A. First Responder Awareness.

   B. First Responder Operations.

   C. Hazardous Materials Technician.

   D. Hazardous Materials Specialist.

ANSWERS

1. **C.**

   The United Nations (UN) number on a diamond placard can be used to identify the substance using the Emergency Response Guidebook.

2. **A.**

   Fixed storage locations for hazardous materials should display a diamond placard with four smaller placards within. Each one provides different information through the use of color, numbers, and symbols.

3. **D.**

   Blue diamond = health hazards; red = fire hazards; yellow = reactivity hazards; white = special hazards.

4. **D.**

   Yellow = reactivity hazards. A number 4 is the highest danger and indicates the potential for spontaneous detonation.

5. **A.**

   Federal law requires EMTs receive First Responder Awareness level training.

Incident Management and Mass Casualty Incidents

I. OVERVIEW OF THE NATIONAL INCIDENT MANAGEMENT SYSTEM (NIMS)

A. NIMS provides an adaptive, standardized approach to any domestic incident.

B. NIMS standardizes the command structure, terminology, training, etc.

C. Standardization allows for effective communication and interaction among multiple and diverse agencies at local, state, and federal levels.

D. The adaptability of NIMS allows it to be used with any type of domestic incident (terrorism, natural disaster, hazardous materials, etc.) of any size.

II. COMPONENTS OF NIMS

A. Preparedness. This component helps agencies and responders proactively prepare for an incident.

B. Communications and Information. This component coordinates effective communication and information sharing.

C. Command and Management. This component provides oversight of the incident for all participating agencies.

D. Resource Management. This component coordinates acquisition, tracking, and recovery of resources and equipment needed during an incident.

E. Ongoing Management. This component coordinates continuous quality improvement of NIMS.

 ## III. NIMS PRACTICES

A. Coordinate efforts through a unified command or single command system to reduce duplication of effort and freelancing.

B. Use "clear text" communications to facilitate interagency efficiency.

C. Limit span of control to no more than seven workers per supervisor.

 ## IV. NIMS ROLE AND RESPONSIBILITIES

A. Command Section. This section includes the incident commander (IC), public information officer (PIO), safety officer, and liaison officer.

B. Finance Section. This section tracks all expenditures during an incident. This section is usually needed only on large incidents.

C. Logistics. The logistics section is responsible for most of the things that actually allow an IMS to function. This includes the necessary communications equipment, medical supplies, food, water, facilities, shelter, etc.

D. Operations. This section is responsible for tactical operations on larger incidents. On smaller incidents, this responsibility usually rests with the IC.

E. Planning. This section helps to develop an action plan for the incident and solve problems as they arise during the incident.

 ## V. EMS FUNCTIONS OF IMS

A. Preparedness

1. EMS agencies should have written disaster plans that are routinely practiced, reviewed, and improved.

2. EMS facilities should have adequate resources to be fully self-sufficient for at least 72 hours.

3. A plan should be in place to assist families of EMS responders so responders can focus on their job.

B. Scene Size-Up

1. What is the incident? Confirm incident location, identify scene safety considerations, estimate number of casualties.

2. What do you need to do? First priorities are personal safety, partner safety, other rescuer's safety, patients' safety, bystanders' and public's safety.

3. What resources do you need to do it? Incident command is established by the highest-ranking person on the scene. Request additional resources as needed.

C. Medical Incident Command Functions

1. Triage

   i. Triage is the sorting of patients based on the severity of injury.

   ii. The triage supervisor identifies the number and severity of patients.

   iii. On larger incidents, several responders may be needed to conduct triage.

   iv. During triage, patients are moved to the appropriate treatment area.

   v. Treatment does *not* begin until all patients are triaged.

2. Treatment

   i. The treatment supervisor establishes the necessary treatment areas based on patient priorities.

   ii. Secondary triage should be completed within each treatment area.

   iii. Treatment area personnel assist with movement of patients to the transportation area.

3. Transportation

   i. The transportation supervisor coordinates transportation of patients to the appropriate destinations.

      ii. Transportation supervisor must ensure receiving hospitals are not overwhelmed.

  4. Staging. The staging supervisor is needed on large incidents when numerous vehicles, agencies, or apparatus will be arriving on the scene.

  5. Rehabilitation. The rehabilitation supervisor establishes a safe location for the rest and recovery of responders. This is typically needed on incidents that are prolonged or work intensive.

  6. Extrication and Special Rescue

      i. An extrication supervisor may be needed on certain incidents.

      ii. The extrication supervisor determines the personnel and equipment needed.

VI. MASS CASUALTY INCIDENTS

A. A mass casualty incident (MCI) is broadly defined as an incident that taxes the locally available resources or requires a multijurisdictional response.

B. Triage Overview

  1. Primary triage

      i. Primary triage is done quickly to determine the patient's basic condition and needs.

      ii. Primary triage is typically done wherever the patient is located.

      iii. The patient's condition is identified through the use of a triage tag and avoids accidental duplication of effort.

  2. Secondary triage. This assessment is done once the patient arrives in the appropriate treatment area.

  3. Triage categories

      i. Immediate

          ➤ Immediate patients are the highest patient priority.

          ➤ Immediate patients have primary assessment problems or exhibit signs and symptoms of head injury or shock.

          ➤ Immediate patients are "red tagged."

    ii. Delayed

       ➤ Delayed patients are the second patient priority.

       ➤ Delayed patients require treatment and transport but not immediately.

       ➤ Delayed patients are "yellow tagged."

    iii. Minor

       ➤ Minor patients are the third patient priority.

       ➤ Delayed patients require little or no treatment by EMS personnel.

       ➤ Delayed patients are also referred to as "walking wounded."

       ➤ Delayed patients are "green tagged."

    iv. Dead or Dying

       ➤ Dead or dying patients are the last patient priority.

       ➤ Also referred to as "expectant" patients because they are either deceased or have a very low chance of survival.

       ➤ Depending on available resources, expectant patients may include cardiac arrest, respiratory arrest, or those with severe head injuries.

       ➤ Expectant patients should be treated only after all other patients have been cared for.

       ➤ Expectant patients are "black tagged."

C. START Triage

  1. Simple Triage and Rapid Treatment (START) was developed in Newport Beach, California, and allows for easy, rapid triage of patients at an MCI.

  2. START triage uses a **RPM** approach to triage by quickly evaluating the patient's **r**espirations, **p**erfusion, and **m**ental status.

  3. START triage step 1

    i. Direct all patients capable of moving to a central location.

    ii. Those able to follow the command and move to the assigned location are collectively triaged as Minor (green tag) or "walking wounded."

4. START triage step 2

   i. Move from patient to patient and begin triage using the RPM method.

     ➤ Respirations

       — If not breathing, manually open the airway. If patient does *not* begin breathing spontaneously, triage as Expectant (black tag) and move to the next patient.

       — If the patient begins to breathe, triage as Immediate (red tag), place in recovery position, and move to next patient.

       — If the patient is breathing spontaneously above 30 breaths per minute or below 10 breaths per minute, triage as Immediate and move to the next patient.

       — If the patient is spontaneously breathing 10 to 30 times per minute, move immediately to the next triage step with that patient.

     ➤ Perfusion

       — Assess radial pulse to determine perfusion status. Avoid assessing the radial pulse on an upper extremity with local trauma that may affect distal circulation in only that extremity.

       — If the radial pulse is absent, triage as Immediate and move to the next patient.

       — If the radial pulse is present, move immediately to the next triage step with that patient.

     ➤ Mental status

       — This is the final step in the RPM triage process and evaluates the patient's ability to follow a simple command.

       — If the patient is unable to follow simple commands, triage as Immediate and move to the next patient.

       — If the patient can follow simple commands, triage as Delayed (yellow tag) and move to the next patient.

5. Special situations

   i. Patients with special needs, such as children, that cannot be triaged effectively with START should be moved as soon as possible to a treatment area for secondary triage.

      ii.   Certain MCIs such as incidents involving hazardous materials or weapons of mass destruction may require additional scene safety precautions such as patient decontamination or law enforcement assistance before triage can occur.

     6. View the START algorithm at *https://chemm.nlm.nih.gov/startadult.htm.*

D. JumpSTART

    1. JumpSTART is for pediatric patients up to 8 years of age.

    2. The JumpSTART algorithm is very similar to the START algorithm, but it is adapted to the physiological differences in children.

      i.   If the pediatric patient is apneic with a palpable pulse, then 5 rescue breaths are attempted. After 5 rescue breaths, spontaneous breathing = IMMEDIATE and continued apnea = DECEASED.

     ii.   Patients with breathing rates less than 15 or over 45 are triaged as IMMEDIATE.

    3. View the JumpSTART algorithm at *https://chemm.nlm.nih.gov/startpediatric.htm.*

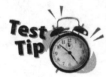

> *For the exam, you need to know the four recognized triage categories and how to sort patients into each of them. Be sure you understand the difference between primary triage and secondary triage.*

PRACTICE QUESTIONS

1. Which of the following provides an adaptive, standardized approach to any domestic mass casualty incident?

   A. NIMS

   B. CISM

   C. SOAP

   D. DNVF

2. During a large incident, NIMS standards require the use of

   A. 10-codes during radio communication.

   B. encoded transmissions for radio communications.

   C. clear text radio communications.

   D. the lead agency's preferred radio codes.

3. On large incidents, the incident commander is part of the

   A. command section.

   B. finance section.

   C. logistics section.

   D. operations section.

4. During a mass casualty incident, comprehensive treatment does NOT begin until

   A. all units arrive on scene.

   B. the incident commander orders it.

   C. the cause of the incident is determined.

   D. all patients have been triaged.

5. During a MCI, when is secondary triage completed?

   A. immediately upon arrival at the scene

   B. once all patients have been counted

   C. once the patient arrives in the treatment area

   D. only if the patient loses consciousness

ANSWERS

1. **A.**

   The National Incident Management System provides an adaptive, standardized approach to domestic incidents.

2. **C.**

   NIMS standards require the use of clear text radio communications.

3. **A.**

   The command section includes the incident commander, public information officer, safety officer, and liaison officer.

4. **D.**

   During an MCI, treatment does not begin until all patients have been triaged.

5. **C.**

   Secondary triage takes place once the patient arrives in the appropriate treatment area.

Terrorism and Weapons of Mass Destruction

I. TERRORIST WEAPONS OF MASS DESTRUCTION (WMD)

A. Scene Safety

1. Your safety is, as always, the first priority during a WMD incident.

2. Follow local protocols and incident command system (ICS) structure regarding response, staging, decontamination, management, and transport of patients during a WMD incident.

B. Explosives

1. Explosives are the most commonly used WMD.

2. Explosive weapons can cause significant blunt and penetrating trauma as well as burns and crushing injuries.

    i.   Primary blast injuries: injuries caused directly by the blast

    ii.   Secondary blast injuries: injuries caused by the flying debris and shrapnel

    iii. Tertiary blast injuries: injuries caused by striking the ground or other objects

C. Chemical Agents

1. Remember that neither extensive training or planning, nor financial resources, are required to develop and use many types of chemical weapons of mass destruction.

2. Nerve agents

    i.   Nerve agents are a significant threat due to the relative ease with which they can be acquired and used.

    ii.   Nerve agents cause excessive parasympathetic nervous system stimulation.

      iii.   Specific nerve agents include Tabun, Sarin, Soman, and VX.

      iv.   Signs and symptoms of nerve agent exposure (**SLUDGEM**)

> **S**alivation, seizures

> **L**acrimation (excessive tearing)

> **U**rination

> **D**efecation

> **G**astric upset

> **E**mesis

> **M**iosis (pupillary constriction)

      v.   Management

> Aggressive airway management, including suction, and ventilatory support may be needed.

> The patient will likely need specific medications to counteract the nerve agent. Get the patient to ALS providers as soon as possible.

3. Vesicants

    i.   Vesicants cause pain, burns, and blisters to exposed skin, eyes, and respiratory tract.

    ii.   Vesicants are also known as blistering agents.

    iii.   Depending on the vesicant agent, the onset of signs and symptoms could be delayed several hours.

    iv.   Affected areas should be irrigated with copious amounts of water as soon as possible.

4. Cyanide

    i.   Cyanide interferes with the body's ability to deliver oxygen to the cells, leading to severe hypoxia and death.

    ii.   Cyanide is also knows as a "blood agent."

    iii.   Signs and symptoms include dizziness, weakness, anxiety, nausea, tachypnea, seizures, and respiratory arrest.

    iv.   Management

> Administer high-flow oxygen.

> Support positive-pressure ventilation as needed.

➤ There are antidotes for cyanide poisoning, but they must be administered quickly by ALS personnel.

5. Pulmonary agents

   i. Pulmonary agents cause lung injury and are also known as "choking agents."

   ii. Signs and symptoms include dyspnea, cough, wheezing, runny nose, and sore throat.

   iii. Management. Manage the airway, administer oxygen, and support ventilations as needed.

6. Biological agents

   i. Biological agents are used to cause disease.

   ii. Even small quantities of certain biological agents can cause disease in a large number of people.

   iii. Signs and symptoms include fever, weakness, respiratory distress, and flu-like symptoms.

   iv. Management is based on providing supportive care for the patient's symptoms.

7. Nuclear and radiological weapons

   i. Nuclear weapons can cause death as a result of the blast, the radiation, or thermal burns.

   ii. Nuclear radiation is dangerous because it can kill living organisms in the body or cause them to mutate. These mutations can lead to birth defects, cancer, and other problems.

   ➤ Alpha radiation

   — Dense, slow-moving radiation. Can travel only short distances.

   — Stopped by clothing, skin, etc., but still very dangerous if patient is contaminated internally, such as through ingestion or inhalation.

   ➤ Beta radiation

   — Slow-moving radiation. Can travel only a few feet.

   — Penetrates only the first few millimeters of skin.

   — Serious risk if patient is internally contaminated through ingestion or inhalation.

➤ Gamma radiation (X-ray)

— Can travel long distances. Easily penetrates the body.

— A significant external hazard risk to living things.

iii. Signs and symptoms of acute radiation sickness include nausea, vomiting, diarrhea, fever, headache, and skin lesions.

iv. Protection from radiation

➤ Time. Spend as little time as possible near a radiation source.

➤ Distance. Get as far away as possible from the radiation source.

➤ Shielding. Gamma radiation will require significant shielding, such as lead or concrete.

v. Management

➤ Consult local protocol regarding decontamination procedures. The patient's clothing or skin could have contaminated debris that is an exposure risk to others. Body fluids of internally contaminated patients are an exposure risk to others.

➤ Remove patients from the source of radiation to a safer location not downwind.

➤ Complete a thorough primary assessment.

➤ Treat blast injuries, tertiary injuries, burn injuries, etc., as you normally would.

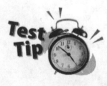

If you would like to learn more about the EMS aspects of terrorism response and WMD, visit https://training.fema.gov/ and take the free online ICS-100 course: Introduction to Incident Command System. Also visit www.teexwmdcampus.com. This website offers a number of online courses certified by the U.S. Department of Homeland Security and the Federal Emergency Management Agency (FEMA). Here are two recommended courses:

AWR111: Basic Concepts for WMD Incidents

AWR160: Terrorism Awareness for Emergency Responders

PRACTICE QUESTIONS

1. What is the most common type of WMD incident?

   A. dirty bomb

   B. biological weapon

   C. explosives

   D. chemical weapon

2. Primary blast injuries are caused by

   A. flying debris and shrapnel.

   B. the blast wave.

   C. striking stationary objects.

   D. penetrating trauma.

3. Death due to massive overstimulation of the parasympathetic nervous system is likely caused by

   A. radiological weapons.

   B. secondary explosives.

   C. biological agents.

   D. nerve agents.

4. SLUDGEM is an acronym designed to help you remember

   A. signs and symptoms of nerve agent exposure.

   B. signs and symptoms of biological agent exposure.

   C. the various types of weapons of mass destruction.

   D. the steps to manage a WMD incident.

5. Vesicants are also known as

   A. sleeping agents.

   B. seizure agents.

   C. nerve agents.

   D. blistering agents.

ANSWERS

1. **C.**

   Explosives are the most common weapon used during a WMD incident.

2. **B.**

   Primary blast injuries are caused by the blast wave.

3. **D.**

   Nerve agents cause massive overstimulation of the parasympathetic nervous system.

4. **A.**

   SLUDGEM is designed to help you remember the signs and symptoms of a nerve agent exposure.

5. **D.**

   Vesicants are blistering agents.

PART VIII
THE PRACTICAL EXAM

The NREMT
Practical Exam

Prior to national certification, the NREMT requires a psychomotor (skills) examination in addition to the computer-based cognitive exam. The process for completing the psychomotor examination varies from state to state. Consult your local EMS office for specifics about completing the psychomotor examination in your state.

The skill sheets that will likely be used or referenced during the psychomotor examination are available at *www.nremt.org*. During the psychomotor examination, candidates may be required to demonstrate competency with any of the following skills:

> ➤ Patient assessment and management of a trauma patient
>
> ➤ Patient assessment and management of a medical patient
>
> ➤ Cardiac arrest management/AED
>
> ➤ Bag valve mask ventilation for an apneic patient
>
> ➤ Spinal immobilization of a supine patient
>
> ➤ Spinal immobilization of a seated patient
>
> ➤ Immobilization of a long-bone fracture
>
> ➤ Immobilization of a joint dislocation
>
> ➤ Traction splinting
>
> ➤ Bleeding control/shock management
>
> ➤ Supplemental oxygen administration

**Top 10 Tips to Prepare
for the Psychomotor Examination**

1. Determine the specifics about the psychomotor examination in your state.

2. Obtain the skill sheets that will be used for your psychomotor exam.

3. Know the skill sheets. Don't just glance at them: read them—review them—know them.

4. Understand the critical actions for each skill. Know the "critical criteria" items that will automatically trigger a retest. These are listed at the bottom of each NREMT skill sheet.

5. Practice! There's no substitute for this. Practice with others who are familiar with the testing process if possible. Practice each skill at least once for each point possible. Example: a 40-point station should be practiced at least 40 times.

6. Determine if the approved training programs in your area offer practice opportunities or other resources to help prepare for the psychomotor examination.

7. Listen carefully to the instructions provided before testing and during each station, including the time limit.

8. If given the opportunity to review or organize your equipment before the station begins, take it!

9. Focus on the current station, not the last station or the next station.

10. Articulate! While testing, do what you say and say what you do. Your hands, mouth, and ears should be busy.

After the Exam

CONGRATULATIONS, you passed your NREMT exam! Welcome to the EMS profession. Now what? Here are the author's top 10 recommendations on what to do next.

#1: CELEBRATE

You have completed an intensive training program and have passed a very difficult comprehensive examination process. You now know better than most that the NREMT only grants EMT certification to those who have earned it. You have demonstrated that you have the knowledge and skills necessary to function competently as a member of the EMS profession. It's time to celebrate! Take a trip, throw a party, or do whatever you can to relax and decompress. Enjoy a break from the rigors of class, homework, tests, etc.

#2: OBTAIN YOUR STATE EMT CERTIFICATION

In most cases, you are not employable as an EMT until you obtain your state certification. The process varies from state to state, but is generally quite simple compared to what you have already accomplished. Most likely you have already received instructions on how to do this during your EMT course. If not, contact your state EMS authority and ask them how to proceed.

#3: UPDATE YOUR RÉSUMÉ

Most professions, including EMS, are moving towards an impersonal, online application process to prescreen job applicants. This means that without a good résumé to precede you, you won't likely get a chance to dress sharp, smile, shake hands, or do any of those other things that make a good first impression. Ask your EMT instructor or another local EMS professional to review your résumé and offer suggestions. There are many good résumé templates available online. To get started, use the sample résumé included at the end of this chapter.

#4: GET A JOB!

What would you like to do with your EMT certification? You could work on an ambulance or rescue unit. You could work in a hospital emergency department or test for the fire department. You could work sporting or concert events or join a search and rescue team. There are, most likely, full-time, part-time, and volunteer EMT opportunities in your community. Hopefully, you had a great EMT classroom instructor; but now it's time for *experience* to be your teacher. There is no substitute for real-life experience. It's time for you to get some!

#5: GEAR UP

Be sure you have the equipment you will need to be ready to go to work. For most new EMTs, that should include a good quality stethoscope; a small, high quality tactical flashlight; and lastly, EMS-related apps for on-call situations.

Author's Note: Please make sure you are up-to-date on all of your immunizations, including the hepatitis-B vaccination series.

#6: JOIN AND READ

EMS is a dynamic profession—the one thing you can count on to stay the same is constant change. Find a way to stay engaged in the profession's "big picture." Consider becoming a member of the National Association of EMTs (NAEMT). NAEMT is a respected national organization focused on issues relevant to EMS professionals. Read the "trade journals." The two most widely recognized periodical publications in the EMS profession are the *Journal of Emergency Medical Services* (JEMS) and *EMS World*. Consider subscribing to at least one of these publications and read them. Both publications include information about job openings around the country and provide access to continuing education opportunities.

#7: ATTEND AN ESM CONFERENCE

Research the availability of local conferences within your area. This is a great way to earn continuing education credits, and network with fellow EMS professionals and employers. Most EMS conferences are buffet style, with multiple break-out sessions happening simultaneously. This allows you to attend the sessions you are most interested in. There are some excellent national EMS conferences, such as the EMS Today Conference, and the EMS World Expo. These annual conferences offer amazing opportunities for learning, networking, and exposure to the latest in EMS equipment and technology.

#8: BEGIN THE RECERTIFICATION PROCESS

About the time you get your EMT certification card in the mail, it's time to start working on your recertification. You have two years before your current certification expires, but the requirements for recertification are extensive. Don't procrastinate! Visit the NREMT website and become familiar with the recertification requirements. Identify local agencies, hospitals, and educational institutions that offer continuing education opportunities. Research various online continuing education opportunities. The NREMT offers some convenient online resources to help track your continuing education and your progress towards meeting the recertification requirements. **CAUTION:** You likely have at least three different expiration dates already. Your CPR certification, state EMT certification, and NREMT certification will likely have different expiration dates. Meeting the recertification requirements is *your* responsibility. Mark your expiration dates on your calendar and set reminders to complete recertification requirements on time.

NOTE: It is much easier to maintain your certifications than it is to get them back once they expire.

#9: DIG DEEPER

Achieving your certification should *not* be considered the end of your learning experience. The best thing now is that you can pick what you would want to learn more about. There are additional certifications available in trauma, pediatric emergencies, medical emergencies, newborn resuscitation, hazardous materials, CPR instructor, and much more. Perhaps there are opportunities for you to become a skills tutor or examiner for a local EMT training program. Consider taking an anatomy and physiology class, pathophysiology class, cardiology or pharmacology class, or something else you are interested in. Ask your EMT instructor for some recommendations.

#10: SAY "THANK YOU"

Thank everyone who helped you. Let your EMT instructor know you passed. Thank your family, friends, employer, coworkers, classmates, mentors, and anyone else that made the journey at least a little easier for you. You will likely lean on some of them again once you decide what the next big challenge will be . . . perhaps paramedic school!

SAMPLE RÉSUMÉ

[Street Address]
[City, ST ZIP Code]
[Telephone]
[Email]

FIRST MIDDLE LAST, NREMT

OBJECTIVE	Employment as an Emergency Medical Technician
SKILLS & ABILITIES	Add something relevant and interesting, such as bilingual
EXPERIENCE	**[JOB TITLE, COMPANY NAME]** [Dates From – To] This is the place for a brief summary of your key responsibilities and most stellar accomplishments.
EDUCATION / CERTIFICATIONS	**ADD COMPLETION OF YOUR EMT COURSE HERE** You might want to include your GPA here and a brief summary of relevant coursework, awards, and honors. **ADD YOUR CPR CERTIFICATION HERE** EX: American Heart Association BLS Healthcare Provider Certification **ADD YOUR STATE EMT CERTIFICATION HERE** EX: EMT certified through the [state] Bureau of Emergency Medical Services. **ADD YOUR NREMT CERTIFICATION HERE** EX: EMT certified through National Registry of Emergency Medical Technicians. **ADD ANY ADDITIONAL CERTIFICATES, DEGREES, ETC. HERE** EX: Online course completion through FEMA Emergency Management Institute.
COMMUNICATION	EX: Strong verbal and written communication skills.
LEADERSHIP	Include leadership experience at work, sports, volunteerism, clubs etc.
REFERENCES	**[REFERENCE NAME]** [Title, Company] [Contact Information]

References

Centers for Disease Control and Prevention (September 2016). Hip fractures among older adults. Retrieved June 3, 2017, from *https://www.cdc.gov/homeandrecreationalsafety/falls/adulthipfx.html*.

Centers for Disease Control and Prevention (October 2016). Suicide prevention. Retrieved June 3, 2017, from *https://www.cdc.gov/violenceprevention/suicide/index.html*.

Federal Emergency Management Agency, U.S. Department of Homeland Security (May 2017). National Incident Management System. Retrieved June 3, 2017, from *https://www.fema.gov/national-incident-management-system*.

Fernandez, A. R., Studnek, J. R., Margolis, G. S. (2008). Estimating the probability of passing the national paramedic certification examination. *Academic Emergency Medicine* 15:258-264.

Hazinski, M., ed. (2010). Highlights of the 2010 American Heart Association guidelines for CPR and ECC. Retrieved June 3, 2017 from *https://www.heart.org/idc/groups/heart-public/@wcm/@ecc/documents/downloadable/ucm_317350.pdf*.

Hettiaratchy, S., Papini, R. (2004). Initial management of a major burn: II—assessment and resuscitation. Retrieved June 3, 2017, from *https://doi.org/10.1136/bmj.329.7457.101*.

Mistovich, J., Keith, K. (2010). *Prehospital emergency care*, 9th ed. Upper Saddle River, NJ: Pearson Education.

National Center for Biotechnology Information, U.S. National Library of Medicine. Pneumothorax. Retrieved June 3, 2017, from *https://www.ncbi.nlm.nih.gov/pubmedhealth/PMHT0023382/*.

National Center for Biotechnology Information, U.S. National Library of Medicine. Sudden infant death syndrome. Retrieved June 3, 2017, from *https://www.ncbi.nlm.nih.gov/pubmedhealth/PMHT0027294/*.

National Center for Biotechnology Information, U.S. National Library of Medicine. Abdominal pain. Retrieved June 3, 2017 from *https://www.ncbi.nlm.nih.gov/pubmedhealth/PMHT0024811/*.

National Center for Biotechnology Information, U.S. National Library of Medicine. Burns. Retrieved June 3, 2017, from *https://www.ncbi.nlm.nih.gov/pubmedhealth/PMHT0027084/*.

National Center for Biotechnology Information, U.S. National Library of Medicine. Heat emergencies. Retrieved June 3, 2017, from *https://medlineplus.gov/ency/article/000056.htm*.

National Center for Biotechnology Information, U.S. National Library of Medicine. Ectopic pregnancy. Retrieved June 3, 2017, from *https://www.ncbi.nlm.nih.gov/pubmedhealth/PMHT0025659/*.

National Center for Biotechnology Information, U.S. National Library of Medicine. Anaphylaxis. Retrieved June 3, 2017, from *https://www.ncbi.nlm.nih.gov/pmc/articles/PMC2954079/*.

National Center for Biotechnology Information, U.S. National Library of Medicine. What is a heart attack. Retrieved June 3, 2017, from *https://www.nhlbi.nih.gov/health/health-topics/topics/heartattack.*

National Center for Biotechnology Information, U.S. National Library of Medicine. Traumatic brain injury. Retrieved June 3, 2017, from *https://www.ninds.nih.gov/disorders/all-disorders/traumatic-brain-injury-information-page.*

National Center for Biotechnology Information, U.S. National Library of Medicine. Seizures. Retrieved June 3, 2017, from *https://www.ncbi.nlm.nih.gov/pubmedhealth/PMHT0023035/.*

National Center for Biotechnology Information, U.S. National Library of Medicine. What is deep vein thrombosis. Retrieved June 3, 2017, from *https://www.nhlbi.nih.gov/health/health-topics/topics/dvt.*

National Center for Biotechnology Information, U.S. National Library of Medicine. Prescription drug abuse. Retrieved June 3, 2017 from *https://medlineplus.gov/prescriptiondrugabuse.html.*

Centers for Disease Control and Prevention (2014). 2014 national diabetes statistics report. Retrieved June 3, 2017 from *https://www.cdc.gov/diabetes/data/statistics/2014statisticsreport.html.*

National Institute of Mental Health. Older adults and depression. Retrieved June 3, 2017 *https://www.nimh.nih.gov/health/publications/older-adults-and-depression/index.shtm*l.

National Registry of Emergency Medical Technicians (n.d.). Cognitive exams general information. Retrieved June 3, 2017, from *https://www.nremt.org/rwd/public/document/cognitive-exam.*

National Registry of Emergency Medical Technicians (2010). 2009 National EMS practice analysis. Columbus, OH: NREMT.

National Registry of EMTs' Implementation of the 2015 AHA Guidelines for CPR and Emergency Cardiovascular Care. Retrieved June 3, 2017, from *https://www.nremt.org/rwd/public/document/news-aha-8-22-16.*

Pollak, A., ed. (2011). *Emergency care and transportation of the sick and injured*, 10th ed. Tall Pine Drive, MA: Jones and Bartlett.

Roach, M. S. (1992). *The human act of caring*. Ottawa, Ontario: Canadian Hospital Association Press.

Rowlett, R., and University of North Carolina at Chapel Hill (July 2001). Glasgow coma scale. Retrieved June 3, 2017, from *http://www.unc.edu/~rowlett/units/scales/glasgow.htm.*

U.S. Department of Health and Human Services, Center for Disease Control (January 2012). Guidelines for field triage of injured patients: recommendations of the national expert panel on field triage, 2011. Retrieved June 3, 2017, from *https://www.cdc.gov/mmwr/preview/mmwrhtml/rr6101a1.htm.*

U.S. Department of Transportation, National Highway Traffic Safety Administration (2009). Emergency medical technician instructional guidelines. Retrieved June 3, 2017, from *http://www.ems.gov/pdf/811077a.pdf.*

U.S. Department of Transportation, National Highway Traffic Safety Administration (2009). National emergency medical services education standards. Retrieved June 3, 2017, from *http://www.ems.gov/pdf/811077a.pdf.*

U.S. National Library of Medicine (September 2014). Actidose. Retrieved June 3, 2017, from *https://dailymed.nlm.nih.gov/dailymed/drugInfo.cfm?setid=61801c3a-caf2-4bb7-a56a-dc2ee007eccb.*

Index